Guiding Adolescents
to Use Healthy Strategies
to Manage Stress

Editors

Kenneth R. Ginsburg, MD, MS Ed, FAAP, FSAHM
Professor of Pediatrics
Perelman School of Medicine at the University of Pennsylvania
Craig-Dalsimer Division of Adolescent Medicine
The Children's Hospital of Philadelphia
Director of Health Services, Covenant House of Pennsylvania
Philadelphia, PA

Sara B. Kinsman, MD, PhD
Associate Professor of Pediatrics
Perelman School of Medicine at the University of Pennsylvania
Craig-Dalsimer Division of Adolescent Medicine
The Children's Hospital of Philadelphia
Philadelphia, PA

American Academy of Pediatrics
141 Northwest Point Blvd
Elk Grove Village, IL 60007-1019

American Academy of Pediatrics Department of Marketing and Publications

Maureen DeRosa, MPA, Director, Department of Marketing and Publications

Mark Grimes, Director, Division of Product Development

Eileen Glasstetter, MS, Manager, Product Development

Mark Ruthman, Manager, Electronic Product Development

Carolyn Kolbaba, Manager, Consumer Publishing

Peter Lynch, Digital Solutions Editor

Amanda Krupa, MSc, CPMW, Editor, Healthy Children.org

Regina Moi, Manager, Patient Education

Mary Claire Walsh, Managing Editor, AAP Web Sites

Sandi King, MS, Director, Division of Publishing and Production Services

Shannan Martin, Publishing and Production Services Specialist

Peg Mulcahy, Manager, Graphic Design and Production

Jason Crase, Manager, Editorial Services

Julia Lee, Director, Division of Marketing and Sales

Linda Smessaert, MSIMC, Brand Manager, Clinical and Professional Publications

Kathleen Juhl, MBA, Manager, Consumer Marketing and Sales

Mary Jo Reynolds, Manager, Consumer Product Marketing

Elyce Goldstein, Manager, Digital Content and Licensing

Sashaya Davis, Institutional Sales Manager

Video Production Team

Mark Ruthman, Producer, American Academy of Pediatrics

Robin Miller, Director and Editor, Robin Miller Videography

Kenneth R. Ginsburg, MD, MS Ed, FAAP, FSAHM, Coproducer, Content Director and Editor

Sara B. Kinsman, MD, PhD, Associate Content Director (Philadelphia)

Colette Auerswald, MD, MS, FSAHM, Associate Content Director (San Francisco)

Arvil Prewitt, Lead Camera Person

Ilana R. Ginsburg, Teen Casting Director

Talia M. Ginsburg, Teen Content Editor

Library of Congress Control Number: 2013948805

ISBN: 978-1-58110-856-9

eISBN: 978-1-58110-857-6

MA0704

The recommendations in this publication do not indicate an exclusive course of treatment or serve as a standard of medical care. Variations, taking into account individual circumstances, may be appropriate.

The American Academy of Pediatrics is not responsible for the content of the resources mentioned in this publication. Web site addresses are as current as possible but may change at any time.

Statements and opinions expressed are those of the authors and not necessarily those of the American Academy of Pediatrics.

Guiding Adolescents to Use Healthy Strategies to Manage Stress is excerpted from *Reaching Teens: Strength-Based Communication Strategies to Build Resilience and Support Healthy Adolescent Development* published by the American Academy of Pediatrics.

Printed in the United States of America.

9-334/0714

2 3 4 5 6 7 8 9 10

Contributors

Marcos O. Almonte, MDiv
Resilience Specialist
El Centro de Estudiantes
Big Picture Philadelphia
Philadelphia, PA

Renata Arrington-Sanders, MD, MPH, ScM, FAAP
Assistant Professor
Division of General Pediatrics and Adolescent
    Medicine
Johns Hopkins School of Medicine
Baltimore, MD

Colette (Coco) Auerswald, MD, MS, FSAHM
Associate Professor
University of California, Berkeley-University of
    California at San Francisco Joint Medical Program
Department of Community Health and Human
    Development
UC, Berkeley School of Public Health
Berkeley, CA

Kenisha Campbell, MD, MPH
Assistant Professor of Pediatrics
Perelman School of Medicine at the University of
    Pennsylvania
Medical Director, Adolescent Primary Care &
    Family Planning
Nicholas and Athena Karabots Pediatric Care Center
Craig-Dalsimer Division of Adolescent Medicine
The Children's Hospital of Philadelphia
Philadelphia, PA

Tonya A. Chaffee, MD, MPH, FAAP
Associate Clinical Professor of Pediatrics
University of California, San Francisco
Director, Teen and Young Adult Health Center
Medical Director, Child and Adolescent Support
    Advocacy and Resource Center
San Francisco General Hospital
San Francisco, CA

Stephanie Contreras
Resilience Specialist
El Centro de Estudiantes
Big Picture Philadelphia
Philadelphia, PA

Alison Culyba, MD, MPH
Fellow, Adolescent Medicine
Craig-Dalsimer Division of Adolescent Medicine
The Children's Hospital of Philadelphia
Philadelphia, PA

Angela Diaz, MD, MPH
Jean C. and James W. Crystal Professor
Departments of Pediatrics and Preventive Medicine
Icahn School of Medicine at Mount Sinai
Director, Mount Sinai Adolescent Health Center
Mount Sinai Hospital
New York, NY

Karyn E. Feit, LCSW
Adolescent Social Worker
Nicholas and Athena Karabots Pediatric Care Center
Family Services, Children's Seashore House
The Children's Hospital of Philadelphia
Philadelphia, PA

Carol A. Ford, MD, FSAHM
Professor of Pediatrics
Perelman School of Medicine at the University
    of Pennsylvania
Chief, Craig-Dalsimer Division of Adolescent
    Medicine
Orton Jackson Endowed Chair in Adolescent
    Medicine
The Children's Hospital of Philadelphia
Philadelphia, PA

Robert Garofalo, MD, MPH
Associate Professor of Pediatrics and Preventive
    Medicine
Northwestern University Feinberg School of
    Medicine
Medical Director, Adolescent HIV Services
Director, Center for Gender, Sexuality and
    HIV Prevention
Ann & Robert H. Lurie Children's Hospital
    of Chicago
Chicago, IL

Kenneth R. Ginsburg, MD, MS Ed, FAAP, FSAHM
Professor of Pediatrics
Perelman School of Medicine at the University
    of Pennsylvania
Craig-Dalsimer Division of Adolescent Medicine
The Children's Hospital of Philadelphia
Director of Health Services, Covenant House
    of Pennsylvania
Philadelphia, PA

Linda A. Hawkins, PhD, LPC
Adolescent Psychotherapist
Adolescent Initiative
Craig-Dalsimer Division of Adolescent Medicine
The Children's Hospital of Philadelphia
Philadelphia, PA

Cordella Hill, MSW
Executive Director
Covenant House Pennsylvania
Philadelphia, PA

Renée R. Jenkins, MD, FAAP
Professor of Pediatrics
Director, Office of Faculty Development
Howard University College of Medicine
Department of Pediatrics and Child Health
Howard University Hospital
Washington, DC

Sara B. Kinsman, MD, PhD
Associate Professor of Clinical Pediatrics
Perelman School of Medicine at the University
    of Pennsylvania
Craig-Dalsimer Division of Adolescent Medicine
The Children's Hospital of Philadelphia
Philadelphia, PA

Richard E. Kreipe, MD, FAAP, FSAHM, FAED
Dr. Elizabeth R. McAnarney Distinguished Professor
of Pediatrics
Division of Adolescent Medicine, Golisano
Children's Hospital
University of Rochester
Medical Director, Western New York Comprehensive
Care Center for Eating Disorders Rochester
Director, New York State ACT for Youth Center
of Excellence
Rochester, NY

LTC Keith M. Lemmon, MD, FAAP
Chief, Division of Adolescent Medicine
Department of Pediatrics
Madigan Army Medical Center
Joint Base Lewis-McChord, WA
Assistant Professor of Pediatrics
Uniformed Services University of the Health Sciences
Bethesda, MD
Clinical Associate Professor of Pediatrics
University of Washington School of Medicine
Seattle, WA

Amanda Lerman, MD
Fellow, Adolescent Medicine
Craig-Dalsimer Division of Adolescent Medicine
The Children's Hospital of Philadelphia
Philadelphia, PA

Joseph Lively
Resilience Specialist
El Centro de Estudiantes
Big Picture Philadelphia
Philadelphia, PA

Hugh Organ, MS
Associate Executive Director
Covenant House Pennsylvania
Chair, Philadelphia Anti-Trafficking Coalition
Philadelphia, PA

Jonathan R. Pletcher, MD, FAAP
Assistant Professor, Pediatrics
University of Pittsburgh School of Medicine
Clinical Director, Division of Adolescent Medicine
Children's Hospital of Pittsburgh of UPMC
Pittsburgh, PA

Daniel H. Reirden, MD, FAAP, AAHIVMS
Assistant Professor of Pediatrics
Sections of Adolescent Medicine and Infectious
Disease
University of Colorado School of Medicine
Medical Director of Youth HIV Services
Children's Hospital Colorado
Aurora, CO

Michael O. Rich, MD, MPH, FAAP, FSAHM
Associate Professor of Pediatrics
Harvard Medical School
Associate Professor of Social and Behavioral
Sciences
Harvard School of Public Health
Director, Center on Media and Child Health
Division of Adolescent Medicine
Boston Children's Hospital
Boston, MA

Nimi Singh, MD, MPH, MA
Assistant Professor, Department of Pediatrics
Division Head, Adolescent Health and Medicine
University of Minnesota Amplatz Children's Hospital
Minneapolis, MN

Jo Ann Sonis, LCSW, DCSW
Licensed Clinical Social Worker
Craig-Dalsimer Division of Adolescent Medicine
Division of Gastroenterology, Hepatology and
Nutrition
The Children's Hospital of Philadelphia
Philadelphia, PA

Susan T. Sugerman, MD, MPH, FAAP
Adolescent Medicine Physician
President and Cofounder
Girls to Women Health and Wellness
Dallas, TX

Dzung X. Vo, MD, FAAP
Assistant Clinical Professor
Division of Adolescent Health and Medicine
Department of Pediatrics
British Columbia Children's Hospital
University of British Columbia
Vancouver, British Columbia
Canada

Zeelyna Wise
Director of Support Services
El Centro de Estudiantes
Big Picture Philadelphia
Philadelphia, PA

Additional Contributors

Several organizations arranged for their young people to participate in this project.

> Covenant House Pennsylvania, Philadelphia, PA
> El Centro de Estudiantes, Philadelphia, PA
> Larkin Street Youth Services, San Francisco, CA
> YouthBuild Philadelphia Charter School,
>   Philadelphia, PA

Professionals from several organizations in the Philadelphia region shared their wisdom in the videos.

Adolescent Advocates, Rosemont, PA
    Ahmed Ghuman, MA
    Sherica Mays-Bankhead, MS, LPC
    Patti Anne McAndrews, MHS, LPC, CAC
    Sean Smith, MEd, AAC I
    Amanda Strittmatter, MSS, LSW, AAC II

Covenant House Pennsylvania, Philadelphia, PA
    Iva Bonaparte
    LuCrecha Coats, MA
    Bianca Cruz
    Carl Hill
    Denise Johnson
    Ciera King
    Pastor David Maddox
    Robert Zindell, MS

El Centro de Estudiantes, Philadelphia, PA
    David Bromley, MS Ed
    Andrew Christman, MA
    Matthew Prochnow, MS Ed
    Helen Rowe, MS Ed
    Tiffaney Whipple, MS Ed

YouthBuild Philadelphia Charter School,
        Philadelphia, PA
    Ameen Akbar
    Ariesha Geier, MS
    Jenee Lee
    Simran Sidhu, MJ

The following individuals contributed to the videos as actors or participants:

Jennie Bernstein
Mei Elansary, MD, MPhil
Stephanie Grossman
Kathryn M. Murphy, RN, PhD
Samantha Powell, MD
Christopher Renjilian, MD
Melissa Riegel
Elyse Salek, MEd
Erin Sieke

Table of Contents

To view the collection of videos and access educational handouts,
please visit www.aap.org/reachingteens/stress.

Introduction ix

**SECTION 1 HOW A STRENGTH-BASED APPROACH AFFECTS
BEHAVIORAL CHANGE** 1

Chapter 1   How a Strength-Based Approach Affects Behavioral Change 3
              Kenneth R. Ginsburg, MD, MS Ed, FAAP, FSAHM

**SECTION 2 THE DEVELOPMENTAL MILIEU AND COMMON STRESSORS
THAT IMPACT TODAY'S TEENS** 7

Chapter 2   The Adolescent World 9
              Amanda Lerman, MD
              Sara B. Kinsman, MD, PhD

Chapter 3   Friendships and Peers...15
              Sara B. Kinsman, MD, PhD

Chapter 4   Perfectionism...27
              Kenneth R. Ginsburg, MD, MS Ed, FAAP, FSAHM
              Susan T. Sugerman, MD, MPH, FAAP

Chapter 5   Grief 35
              Alison Culyba, MD, MPH
              Sara B. Kinsman, MD, PhD

SECTION 3 STRATEGIES TO HELP YOUTH COPE WITH CHALLENGES 47

Chapter 6   Health Realization—Accessing a Higher State of Mind
              No Matter What..49
              Nimi Singh, MD, MPH, MA

Chapter 7   The Role of Lifestyle in Mental Health Promotion 55
              Nimi Singh, MD, MPH, MA

Chapter 8   Stress Management and Coping...61
              Kenneth R. Ginsburg, MD, MS Ed, FAAP, FSAHM

Chapter 9   Mindfulness Practice for Resilience and Managing Stress and Pain.............71
              Dzung X. Vo, MD, FAAP

**SECTION 4 APPROACHES TO REACH YOUTH AND FACILITATE
POSITIVE CHANGE** 79

Chapter 10   Addressing Demoralization: Eliciting and Reflecting Strengths 81
              Kenneth R. Ginsburg, MD, MS Ed, FAAP, FSAHM

Chapter 11   Motivational Interviewing 87
              Nimi Singh, MD, MPH, MA

**SECTION 5 STRATEGIES TO HELP ADOLESCENTS OWN
THEIR SOLUTIONS** 97

Chapter 12   Helping Adolescents Own Their Solutions 99
              Kenneth R. Ginsburg, MD, MS Ed, FAAP, FSAHM

Chapter 13   Gaining a Sense of Control—One Step at a Time....................................105
              Kenneth R. Ginsburg, MD, MS Ed, FAAP, FSAHM

**SECTION 6 DELIVERING BAD NEWS IN A WAY THAT MAY
BUFFER INEVITABLE STRESS** 111

Chapter 14   Delivering Bad News to Adolescents..113
              Daniel H. Reirden, MD, FAAP, AAHIVMS
              Kenneth R. Ginsburg, MD, MS Ed, FAAP, FSAHM

SECTION 7 DE-ESCALATION AND CRISIS MANAGEMENT STRATEGIES.............. 119

Chapter 15   De-escalation and Crisis Management When a Youth Is "Acting Out" 121
              Cordella Hill, MSW
              Hugh Organ, MS
              Kenneth R. Ginsburg, MD, MS Ed, FAAP, FSAHM

INDEX 129

Introduction

We all recognize how real stress can be. In today's pressure-cooker society, youth need to tap into their strengths, acquire specific skills to cope, recover from adversity, and be prepared for future challenges. That's a tall order for all young people but may be particularly challenging for youth who are exposed to chronic stress or traumatic experiences.

Most risky adolescent behaviors serve at least partly as coping strategies that help youth manage uncomfortable stressors. These behaviors offer fleeting relief but lead to troubling patterns that only magnify stress and are in some cases life threatening. If we help youth develop a range of alternative coping strategies, we will diminish their need to turn to these worrisome quick fixes.

Developed for all youth-serving professionals, *Guiding Adolescents to Use Healthy Strategies to Manage Stress* reviews the basic principles of strength-based communication, discusses the sources of worry for teens, offers practical approaches for helping youth understand they can control their reactions and behaviors, and offers us strategies to de-escalate tension when stressors lead to crises.

(This content focusing on stress is excerpted from a much larger body of work, *Reaching Teens: Strength-Based Communication Strategies to Build Resilience and Support Healthy Adolescent Development* [www.aap.org/reachingteens].)

■ Why Focus on Adolescents?

Adolescence is a time of great promise and potential when each young person strives to answer the fundamental question, "Who am I?" It is the stage when youth are learning to navigate their environment, imagining what independence may look like, and considering how they might contribute to the world. It is the time when teens begin to explore intimate relationships that will hopefully lead to them having healthy and satisfying adult lives.

Although adolescence is a time of inspirational possibility, it is also a stage of potential peril. Teens struggle to individuate from their parents and discover how they are just like—and so very different from—them. This can lead to rebellion. Peers take on a pivotal importance as young people try on different personas and experiment with new behaviors. For these reasons among others, the greatest threats to adolescents' lives and well-being are tightly linked to their behavior.

The Teen Years Are the Time When Healthy and Dangerous Lifelong Habits Are Formed

Adolescence is often framed as a time of fierce independence when adult guidance is rejected. In fact, adolescents are hungry for guidance. Although parents are ideally situated to offer their wisdom and experience, they are also the people from whom youth are programmed to wrest independence. This means that youth-serving professionals have a crucial role in guiding teens to make the choices that will position them to thrive now and into adulthood and in supporting parents to optimize their influence.

■ Our Philosophical Framework

There are several core principles drawn largely from the positive youth development and resilience frameworks that guide this work.
- While we hope youth will avoid risk behaviors, our goal is to prepare them to thrive and to position them to be fully prepared to lead us into the future.
- Youth have inherent strengths to be recognized and developed, and the best way to address risk may be to build on these existing strengths.

- Young people need to feel valued. They need to know that they matter. When adults genuinely listen to their views and recognize that they are the experts on their own lives, it empowers them to make healthy decisions.
- Youth thrive when they have strong healthy connections with adults who believe in them unconditionally and hold them to high expectations. Ideally, youth have those connections with their parents. When they do, healthy connections with other adults expand that protection. When they don't, healthy connections with other adults take on a critical importance.
- Ideally, healthy development is supported from early in infancy. When it is not, adolescents are still capable of healing and do so best when caring adults trust in their capacity to right themselves and offer appropriate support and guidance.
- Most risky adolescent behaviors (including substance use, self-mutilation, violence, Internet addiction, and a host of other problems) serve at least partly as coping strategies that help youth manage uncomfortable stressors. If we help youth to develop a repertoire of alternative coping strategies, we will diminish their need to turn to these worrisome quick fixes.
- When we work with youth who have experienced trauma and are exhibiting acting-out behaviors, it is important to approach them with the unspoken mindset of "What happened to you?" rather than "What's wrong with you?" In fact, because trauma is so prevalent and we never know someone's full past, it is wise to approach all youth with this nonjudgmental, supportive mind-set.

The overarching goal of *Reaching Teens* is to enhance your comfort and skill in communicating with teenagers so that you are better positioned to guide them. The specific goal of *Guiding Adolescents to Use Healthy Strategies to Manage Stress* is to build your skill sets in helping adolescents manage life's challenges in a healthy manner while making wise decisions. Therefore, it offers basic principles of strength-based, trauma-informed communication; approaches to connect with youth; and specific strategies and brief interventions to deal with issues likely to arise as you serve adolescents and their families.

The written word is not the most natural way to convey concepts in communication. Therefore, although strategies are anchored in written chapters, video materials allow for deeper explanations, alternate views, youth input, and demonstrations. These materials can be accessed through www.aap.org/reachingteens/stress.

Reaching Teens knows you are the expert on your own practice. It does not suggest replacing your style with any approach offered here; rather, it offers a repertoire of strategies you may choose from to supplement your own. In fact, you will note intentional redundancy where different experts may cover the same topic and at times may even offer conflicting views.

■ Informed by the Best Available Evidence

This work draws from the best of existing evidence to develop applied, theoretically based communication strategies. It is important, however, to understand that many of the techniques shared in this work have not been formally studied and therefore do not meet the highest standards of evidence. We hope that researchers dive deeply into how best to engage teens; however, the current literature is scant and much of what we believe involves difficult-to-study constructs. For example, a wide body of research demonstrates that a sense of connection with positive adults and peers is a core element that determines a young person's well-being. However, there is not a literature that clearly evaluates the varied ways in which to forge connections. Part of the reason this literature is sparse is because of how difficult it is to truly measure the essential ingredients of connection, such as trust, respect, and positive regard. In fact, we recognize many of these concepts are even difficult to clearly define.

In a subject area steeped in the nuances of human interactions, we choose not to be limited by the standards of being research-based but will consistently be informed by the best of existing evidence, including expert opinion. Further, we are rooted in the theoretical constructs of the positive youth development and resilience movements.

Continuing Education and Building a Better Practice

This work is not designed to teach you to do therapy; rather, it hopes to enhance your already existing therapeutic skills. Communication skills are built over a lifetime of service, with each interaction offering a new challenge and opportunity for growth. If you do not occasionally struggle with issues around communication, you are not human. The key to continued growth is practice, self-reflection, and safe and ongoing feedback. We believe that some of the best feedback can come from our colleagues who are invested in our ongoing growth as well as career longevity.

Each chapter will offer questions in a section called "Group Learning and Discussion" so that you can work with your colleagues to take a deeper dive and consider how the lessons best apply to the youth you serve. Ideally, your group can use this for quality improvement within your practice. Continuing education credits are offered through the work *Reaching Teens*.

Trust

As you consider adding new strategies to your communications repertoire, it is important to know that you will be fitting them on for size and will likely have varying levels of success. No strategy works for all youth, which is why it is so helpful to have a variety of approaches from which you can draw. Please do trust, however, that when you use a strength-based approach, at the very least you are empowering teens to make good decisions, even if the outcomes are not clearly evident to you at the moment.

■ The Content

Guiding Adolescents is divided into 7 sections; videos (accessed through www.aap.org/reachingteens/stress) accompany each chapter to allow for deeper explanations, youth input, and demonstrations.

Section 1—How a Strength-Based Approach Affects Behavioral Change

Our overriding goal is to guide youth toward health-affirming behaviors and wise decisions. Telling them what not to do can backfire, whereas building on existing strengths positions them as the experts in their lives and therefore facilitates positive behavioral change (Chapter 1).

Section 2—The Developmental Milieu and Common Stressors That Impact Today's Teens

Chapter 2, "The Adolescent World," reminds us of the complexities of growing up today. In sharp contrast to viewing adolescence as carefree years, we must understand how stressful navigating the teen years can be. Among these stresses are the constant pushing and pulling, the joys and agonies, of interacting with peers, discussed in Chapter 3. For some of our youth, the desire to succeed in an ever-more competitive world, combined with pressures from schools, families, and friends, lead to perfectionism, which is discussed in Chapter 4. Finally, Chapter 5, "Grief," considers the impact of these extreme circumstances on the well-being of youth.

Section 3—Strategies to Help Youth Cope With Challenges

The impact of stressful events in our lives is not inevitable; it is highly influenced by our general state of physical and emotional health, our belief in our ability to "right" ourselves, how we perceive stressors, and the strategies we use to manage them. Chapter 6, the health realization model, sets the tone for this section by elucidating the self-righting tools each of us possess to return to a state of balance. In Chapter 7, the critical role of a healthy lifestyle is underscored. Chapter 8 offers a comprehensive strategy to help young people manage stress healthfully. It starts with how they choose to evaluate stressors and then offers a toolbox that young people (starting early in childhood) can use to manage their emotions and problems. It also offers positive strategies that allow a young person to disengage healthfully. When youth do not possess healthy disengagement strategies, they may seek substances that help them to zone out. Much of our stress and suffering comes from being pulled away from the present moment. Our minds may be caught in regrets about the past, worries about the future, or judgments about the present. Mindfulness practice (Chapter 9) allows one to be fully present with kindness and without judgment (toward self and others).

Section 4—Approaches to Reach Youth and Facilitate Positive Change

A critical step to helping teens manage stress is to give them a sense of control over their destiny. Demoralization, hopelessness, and helplessness drive youth toward dangerous solutions that avoid problems or make them feel better for a moment. Demoralized youth do not believe in their potential to change, leaving them feeling powerless and out of control. A critical first step, discussed in Chapter 10, is to always address risk in the clear context of seeing youths' strengths. When we do this, we help them understand that we view them positively and reinforce that they are deserving and capable of change. Motivational interviewing (Chapter 11) is a well-researched method that gives youth control over their own behaviors and decisions. It positions youth as the experts and ultimate decision-makers and professionals as facilitators.

Section 5—Strategies to Help Adolescents Own Their Solutions

Youth who are stressed or in crisis often cannot clearly think through situations. They may metaphorically view problems as "mountains" too large to overcome. Their inability to break problems down into manageable components ("hills") prevents their progress, magnifies their stress, and often leads to decisions that have not been wisely considered. Further, when we try to guide youth in a manner they cannot comprehend (eg, lecturing an adolescent who is in crisis or not yet cognitively equipped to consider abstract logic), we add to their sense of powerlessness and stress. In Chapter 12, we will discuss how to help adolescents arrive at and therefore "own" their solutions by facilitating their thought processes using concrete communication strategies. Chapter 13 will offer another technique that helps youth move forward by learning to traverse one "hill" at a time, thereby making the summit of the mountain feel within reach.

Section 6—Delivering Bad News in a Way That May Buffer Inevitable Stress

Youth are often in crisis because of a potentially life-changing circumstance. We professionals are often the bearer of "bad news" ranging from pregnancy to knowledge of a family tragedy to a medical diagnosis. Although we can't eliminate the stress associated with these disclosures, our delivery style can buffer the associated shock or trauma (Chapter 14).

Section 7—De-escalation and Crisis Management Strategies

Sometimes youth internalize stress with depression or withdrawal; other times they act out with rage. In Chapter 15, youth-serving agencies offer wisdom on managing and de-escalating crises.

How a Strength-Based Approach Affects Behavioral Change

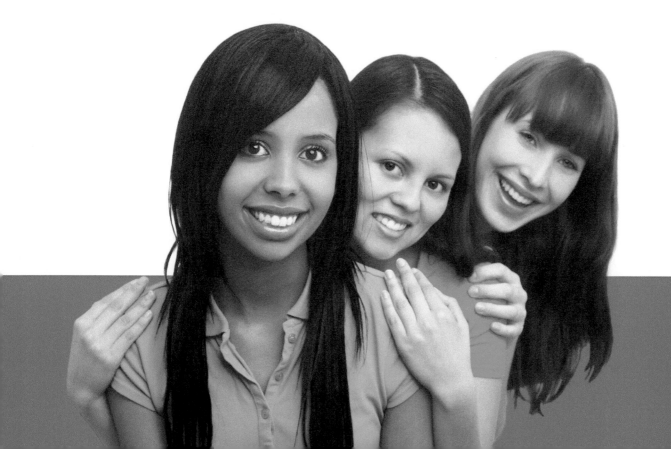

CHAPTER 1

How a Strength-Based Approach Affects Behavioral Change

Kenneth R. Ginsburg, MD, MS Ed, FAAP, FSAHM

 Related Video Content

1.0 How a Strength-Based Approach Supports Behavioral Change

■ Why This Matters

Adolescent health and well-being are largely determined by behaviors. In fact, nearly 80% of mortality is behaviorally related and a substantial amount of morbidity is associated with emotional health and behavioral decisions.

The impact of encouraging positive behavioral choices during adolescence reaches far beyond the teen years. Thinking patterns formed in adolescence may persist and affect adult emotional well-being. Many behaviors that deeply affect health (eg, cigarette use and other addictions, sexual habits) may begin in adolescence, and many health habits (eg, exercise, nutrition, appropriate sleep, relaxation strategies) that will heavily influence physical and emotional health begin in adolescence.

Our role in helping young people make and sustain healthy choices affects health far into the future.

The strength-based interviewing and assessment techniques suggested throughout much of this textbook are designed to support positive behavioral change by forging connections, building confidence, and fostering motivation. Similarly, some of the skills discussed, such as developing positive coping strategies or solving problems one step at a time, reinforce positive behavioral decisions.

> **Many habits and behaviors that will heavily influence lifelong physical and emotional health begin in adolescence. Therefore, the impact of encouraging positive behavioral choices during adolescence reaches far beyond the teen years.**

■ Stages of Behavioral Change

Behavioral changes are not usually "events," rather they are active or passive decisions made over time that can be supported or undermined by life circumstances, media, peers, family, and helping professionals.

The process of behavioral change is posited in many different theoretical frameworks, but Prochaska's transtheoretical model of behavioral change (TTM) is a helpful tool to conceptualize this process in adolescents.[1] The TTM suggests that individuals proceed through a series of stages as they attempt to change aspects of their lives, and it offers important insights into the factors that inhibit or promote positive change at each stage. The TTM predicts youth progress through the following stages of change:

1. Precontemplation (youth has no intention of changing or denies need for change)
2. Contemplation (youth is considering change and weighing perceived costs and benefits)
3. Preparation (youth is actively planning to change)
4. Action (youth is making an attempt to change)
5. Maintenance (youth is solidifying change and resisting relapse)

One of the key concepts within TTM is decisional balance. This involves a weighing of costs and benefits, or pros and cons of any behavior.[2] The relative weight of the pros and cons helps determine a person's readiness to move forward in the behavioral change process. If the perceived benefits (pros) of a behavior outweigh the perceived costs (cons), it may make no sense to a person to consider thinking about change (ie, she will not move beyond precontemplation). She moves toward contemplation when the decisional balance is more even, and is ready for action when the cons of the behavior are seen as outweighing the benefits. A person will likely only maintain a new behavior when the benefits of the new healthy behavior consistently outweigh the perceived benefits of the replaced behavior. One can assess an individual's progress through these stages not only by tracking behavior, but also by evaluating changes in confidence and in relative weighting of the costs and benefits of change.

A youth may be at a different stage of change for various behaviors. Interactions can be most effective if the stage of change is identified for the targeted behavior and appropriate information and support is offered to move the young person toward the next stage.[3] At the earlier stages, awareness of the causes and consequences of a behavior, or the perception of available alternatives, can influence an individual's progress.[4] But forward movement can be paralyzed by a person's belief that he is incapable or unworthy of change. Once a person has decided to move forward, it is critical that he has the skills to do so, because a motivated person who lacks skills will find frustration. Some of those skills should involve adaptive behaviors to replace the benefit of the old behaviors. Further, if a person is to maintain a behavior, support and reinforcement from others can be important, and the skills to resist pressure to return to destructive behaviors may be critical.

■ Adjusting Interaction Approach Based on Stage of Change

An assessment that includes an area to be addressed as well as a stage of behavioral change allows us to better hone our interactions.

- During *precontemplation*, the young person may be unaware of a problem altogether, not grasp the consequences of her behavior, or be demoralized about her ability to change. At this stage, it is important to both give information and build confidence if needed. It makes sense also to get an idea of what benefits and costs the adolescent sees in her current behavior.
- During *contemplation*, the young person is beginning to consider change and determining if the change is likely to be worthwhile. We may be most effective by helping the youth understand the benefits of alternative behaviors. It is also important to help her gain the confidence to believe that if she takes positive action, she will likely succeed. This may be an opportune time to begin introducing skills.
- During *preparation*, the young person is seriously considering taking action. It is particularly important here that she is equipped with appropriate skills. No matter the level of motivation, the change process will fail without the concrete skills (eg, getting condoms, knowing how to put them on) and negotiation skills (eg, dealing with partners who say condoms are not natural) a youth needs to be able to put her plans into operation.

- When an adolescent has decided to take *action,* it is particularly important that negative learned behaviors are replaced with positive ones. Because many behaviors have effectively reduced stress, the adolescent needs positive strategies that also ameliorate stress. Otherwise, the decisional balance will weigh in favor of the former behavior.
- If the teen has already tried out new behaviors and is trying hard to *maintain* those behaviors, it is important that positive reinforcement comes from parents, peers, and you. Without this reinforcement, the adolescent may relapse in response to negative influence or long-held low expectations or critical self-appraisal. Here might be the time to reassess pressures that may be destructive and reinforce the navigational skills that will allow her to continue forward movement.

■ Reaching Teens: Infused With Strength-Based Strategies Designed to Promote Positive Behavioral Change

Many strength-based techniques included throughout this work hold the potential to promote positive change. As you consider each technique suggested throughout this text, it may be helpful to consider how it could reinforce your ability to promote positive change. A few examples are offered here.

Strategies That Position You to Be an Agent of Change

- *Setting the Stage for Trustworthy Interactions:* This strategy builds the type of relationship where an adolescent and family consider a professional trustworthy enough to be an ally in the behavioral change process (see *Reaching Teens*).
- *Understanding Youth Are Experts in Their Own Lives:* Our goal is to influence youth behavior, not to impose our views. Adolescence is a time where the developmental imperative is answering the question, "Who am I?" Therefore, having a sense of control over their decisions and views is essential. When they feel controlled they rebel. When we value the expertise they have, they may invite us into their lives. When we acknowledge that only they have the wisdom and experience to know how to navigate their own circumstances, they will be more likely to join with us to consider how to move forward (see *Reaching Teens*).
- *Eliciting and Reflecting Strengths:* This technique focuses on building a teen's confidence in his belief that he can change. It is particularly useful for teens who may be demoralized or who see themselves as powerless or unworthy to initiate change (see Chapter 10).
- *Motivational Interviewing:* This method facilitates an adolescent to consider the pros and cons of a given behavior in order to develop discrepancy between her current behaviors and goals. The entire premise is to move adolescents toward positive behavioral change (see Chapter 11).
- *Circle of Courage:* This approach is another technique that elicits, reflects, and builds strengths while exploring 4 key youth assets: Mastery, Belonging, Independence, and Generosity (see *Reaching Teens*).

Strategies That Offer Strength-Building Skills

- *Social Skills to Navigate Peer Culture:* If a youth has decided to choose positive behaviors and activities, but his peer group has not, his decisional balance will likely weigh against positive movement (ie, being good vs losing friends). If he is equipped with skills that allow him both to make healthy choices *and* successfully navigate peer culture, he is more likely to initially take action and maintain the positive behaviors, even in the face of pressure to revert to old behaviors (see Chapter 3).

- *Reinforcing Parental Strategies for Effective Discipline and Monitoring:* Young people become demoralized when they see no connection between their action and consequences. Youth who feel "controlled" learn that their choices don't matter. Parents who know how to appropriately discipline teach children that their behavior leads to consequences; good behavior leads to rewards and increasing freedoms and responsibility while poor behavior requires parents to tighten the reins out of concern for safety. Youth who understand that the choices they make matter may be more likely to choose their behaviors wisely (see *Reaching Teens*).
- *Taking Control—One Step at a Time:* A young person can want to do the right thing but become demoralized as she considers how overwhelming the process of change may be. This will cost her the needed confidence to even contemplate change. If she is facilitated to break the process of change into smaller component parts, she may achieve a better sense of control over her choices (see Chapter 13).
- *Mindfulness:* Young people can become stuck in the stories of their past or paralyzed as they contemplate their future. This can prevent them from conserving the energy needed to take action in the present (see Chapter 9).
- *Positive Coping Strategies:* Because many worrisome behaviors reduce stress, a young person needs effective positive strategies that also lower stress. Otherwise, the social risks will continue to offer very real benefits that outweigh the costs. In primary prevention, youth develop a repertoire of activities and skill sets that serve as positive stress-reduction strategies. In secondary prevention, an adolescent already engaging in a negative behavior is guided to build positive coping strategies. A person with existing positive strategies may never "learn" the benefit of negative quick fixes. A person using negative behaviors for stress reduction may shift her decisional balance if positive behaviors consistently offer relief (see Chapter 8).

●● Group Learning and Discussion ●●

This chapter serves as a "landing page" for a variety of behavioral change strategies. Your group should have a general discussion on how to adjust interaction style based on stage of behavioral change. Then you should focus on one of the specific strategies to build your skills.

■ References

1. Prochaska JO. Decision making in the transtheoretical model of behavior change. *Med Decis Making.* 2008;28(6):845–849
2. Velicer WF, Prochaska JO, Fava JL, Norman GJ, Redding CA. Smoking cessation and stress management: applications of the transtheoretical model of behavior change. *Homeost.* 1998;38:216–233
3. Prochaska JO, Velicer WF. The transtheoretical model of health behavior change. *Am J Health Promot.* 1997;12:38–48
4. Prochaska JO, DiClemente CC, Norcross JC. In search of how people change. Applications to addictive behaviors. *Am Psychol.* 1992;47(9):1102–1114

■ Related Video Content

1.0 How a Strength-Based Approach Supports Behavioral Change. Ginsburg.

1.1 The Second Decade of Life Impacts Health and Well-being Over the Life Span. Ford, Auerswald, Diaz, Jenkins.

The Developmental Milieu and Common Stressors That Impact Today's Teens

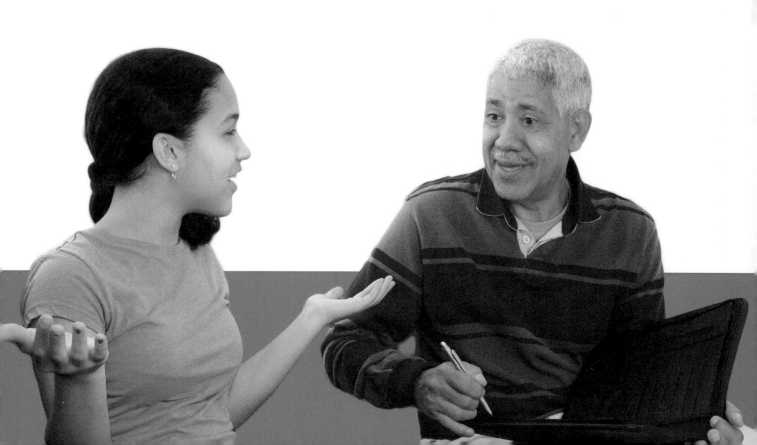

CHAPTER 2

The Adolescent World

Amanda Lerman, MD
Sara B. Kinsman, MD, PhD

■ Why This Matters

Some adults regard young people as living in an easygoing world free of serious responsibility. Their basic needs are often still provided by adults, and they seem to spend their time in unproductive ways: hanging out, watching TV, playing games, and messaging each other minute-to-minute. Parents, teachers, and other adults marvel at how much time teenagers expend in seemingly inconsequential activity. They may continually ask, "What did you do with the whole day?" More than likely, adolescents will not be able to explain fully what they "accomplished," and their uninformative responses may further the adult's view that teens "waste time" in trivial activities. Similarly, adults often struggle to understand how adolescents can get so concerned, excited, or upset over seemingly small matters. Bewildered, they may blame hormones.

> **Adults have all been through childhood and adolescence, and their own memories may be helpful in relating to young people. Personal experience, though, can grant a false sense of complete understanding. The adolescent world has challenges that adults have forgotten about, play down, or even repress.**

It can be hard as an adult to see young people's world through their lens. In her 1988 novel, *Cat's Eye,* which explored relationships between female childhood friends, Margret Atwood illustrates this phenomenon, writing:

> "Little girls are cute and small only to adults. To one another they are not cute. They are life-sized."[1]

Adults have all been through childhood and adolescence, and their own memories may be helpful in relating to young people. Personal experience, though, can grant a false sense of complete understanding. The adolescent world has challenges that adults have forgotten about, play down, or even repress. Still few adults would voluntarily step back in life to relive the joy of middle school. Remembering the very real challenges that come with transitioning from childhood to adulthood can help us better understand and empathize with the ways adolescents negotiate their world.

■ Activities, Interests, and Identity Formation

Just as little children need time to play and learn about their world,[2] the unstructured time spent by adolescents is critically important for their social development. Adolescents need to explore their world and their place in it. When they spend hours "hanging out" with people their own age, they are learning how to communicate with peers and develop social skills. This is a time of trial and error. Adolescents learn that they cannot control their friends' comments or behaviors and that unlike most family members, classmates are not always interested in being fair, kind, or supportive. Meanwhile, most adolescents start to identify attributes in peers who are "good matches"; recognizing these qualities can guide them toward the people their age who can become enduring and reliable friends and extend their social world beyond the family.

Other activities also irk parents. They worry about excessive time and energy spent changing clothes, perfecting hairstyles, and scrutinizing their bodies. When young people obsess over their physical appearances, though, they are not being shallow—they are beginning to think about how they present themselves to the world. They are trying on different identities to see what is comfortable and what feels "like me." When teenagers develop keen interest in idols—celebrities, actors, musicians, sports stars—they are not just mimicking pop culture, they are aligning themselves with different role models to see how they fit. When youth jump from one activity to another, they are not necessarily "quitters"; they may be exploring their various abilities. When adolescents join subcultures—musical subcultures like goth, punk, or hip hop; lifestyle subcultures like vegan or gamer, or, in past years, hippie; or fraternities, sororities, clubs, or other groups—they are not just blindly following or seeking acceptance, they are also trying on identities as they search for their true selves. All of these endeavors may seem frivolous to adults, but they present adolescents with opportunities to create, problem solve, and develop in multiple ways. What seems a waste of time to some adults may actually be critical to youth development, since even more daunting than figuring out the external world is discovering one's own identity.

The focus on the external—appearance, image, and association—can make these pursuits appear useless, misguided, or even harmful, but the surface is simply the easiest place to start. Initial attempts toward defining and redesigning their public face may represent the first move teens make from a passive sense of self based on predetermined characteristics (such as biological sex or skin color) toward active identity formation. Deeper introspection, self-adjustment, and growth can follow.

Similarly, young people do not just investigate and assimilate existing culture—they play an active role in reinventing it. Children and adolescents have long been regarded as being "socialized" by the world in which they are raised, but there is now evidence that this process is not unidirectional. Sociologists have observed that growing minds do not just absorb and mirror the culture they experience—they appropriate and reshape it.[3] Adolescents are molded by their world, and they in turn rearrange the cultures they encounter. We all see examples of this every day. Young minds create most new language—slang, which ultimately becomes canonized in the *Oxford English Dictionary*. Young hearts have fueled societal change throughout history: consider their role in the French Revolution or the American civil rights movement. Young people challenge adults not because they are hormone-crazed, irrational, or delinquent, but because they see novel solutions, embrace change, and fight for progress even when it requires upheaval of the current order.

■ More Difficult Than You May Remember

The lives of adolescents may not involve many bills to pay, but they contain an enormous amount of uncertainty and can include overwhelming stress. Some youth endure significant hardships such as bullying, abuse, abandonment, poverty, homelessness, and other life-threatening adversities. Others struggle with mental or physical illness. We can readily feel for teens who are visibly suffering, but it is not always clear when young people are in distress. The warning signs that an adolescent is hurting can be subtle or simply different from what we might expect. Adolescents struggling with major depression, for example, may display the profound sadness seen in depressed adults. Unlike adults, however, they are just as likely to exhibit irritability, or even rage, as the main symptom of depression. This can evoke our anger rather than our support.

Teens may be embarrassed or ashamed to reveal their pain, may struggle to put their feelings into words, or may have no idea what they are experiencing. If young people do not respond when asked "What's wrong?" it may be because they have no answer to the question.

The most disadvantaged youth, who may have the greatest need, may also be the most easily misunderstood. Some grow up lacking basic necessities and may see no reason to hope for a better life. As compassionate citizens, we lament the substandard education provided by their underfunded schools, the tragic shortcomings of the foster care system, or their inconsistent access to quality health care, but our concern may not be apparent to them. They may notice instead the uneasiness they inspire in other people in stores, on the street, or on public transit. The greatest obstacle to meeting their potential may be when they internalize these low expectations.

The challenges of adolescence are not limited to the sickest, most troubled, or most disadvantaged teens. The stress of this transitional period can be oppressive to youth in any setting. Even if an adolescent does not directly experience hardship, they know of others who have and have become aware of the unfairness of suffering. These realizations are unsettling as an individual transforms from viewing the world as a child to holding the more complex worldview of adults.

Struggling to make sense of the world's harsh realities can be terrifying, especially since modest life experience makes it hard to recognize all its possibilities. The classic 1986 film *Stand By Me* sensitively captures the unmitigated feelings of youthful inexperience. It tells the tale of a formative weekend expedition embarked upon by 4 young friends in late summer before starting junior high school. The main character narrates the tale from adulthood. As the picture opens, he explains:

> "I was living in a small town in Oregon called Castle Rock. There were only twelve hundred and eighty-one people. But to me, it was the whole world."[4]

Seen through the frame of a man in middle age reflecting and redefining his experiences as a 12-year-old boy, the emotional moments in the picture are far more poignant. As he recounts the plot, the narrator implicitly tells the story of youthful innocence, reminding audiences what it actually felt like to be young, inexperienced, and unaware of the size of the world beyond a small town. Decades later it can be near impossible to conjure up that feeling, to un-know what one now knows and remember how real teenage anxieties and heartaches felt. With a limited view of the world at large, every problem can loom large—each family quarrel can seem insurmountable, each test can threaten to determine lifetime potential for success or failure, and each interpersonal conflict can forebode a lifetime of social rejection.

Columnist Dan Savage's "It Gets Better" Web video campaign, created in 2010 to "show young LGBT people the levels of happiness, potential, and positivity their lives will reach—if they can just get through their teen years,"[5] highlights the truncated perspective that all teenagers experience. The movement features videos created by lesbian, gay, bisexual, and transgendered (LGBT) adults reflecting on the difficulties of their teen years and telling the hopeful tales of how much better their lives became after adolescence—after graduating from the high schools that circumscribed their social experiences, after gaining independence from judgmental family units, after moving on from intolerant home communities. The lesson on perspective, created specifically to address the particularly intense isolation frequently experienced by LGBT youth, can be extended to all young people. The worlds of adolescents are limited. Without broader outlook, the bullying, judgment, or condemnation of a few individuals can seem like rejection by the whole world, and, without greater context, everyday pressures can be crushing.

Clearly not every young person struggles with sexual orientation, or with bullying, but they all have different and unique challenges. Adolescent worlds exist in infinite varieties representing the brilliant diversity of young people, but they are all constrained by a short lifetime of previous experiences. As they emerge from childhood into an awareness of the complexity of the world, young people know that they have only a few years before they have to navigate it independently. In the best situations, teenagers have adults around them that empower them to find their own dreams and encourage them to excel, but the broad array of possibilities can be dizzying. If adults are not careful with their messages, it can seem to young people that any misstep could be catastrophic.

■ Here's What to Do

As new members of society, adolescents are charged with the task of making sense of the world around them and, even more daunting, with figuring out how they fit into it. Rather than fearing their potential for innovation, we can foster it. Young people are not yet vastly experienced in the world, but they have a tremendous amount to contribute. When we make assumptions about adolescents' thoughts, feelings, and experiences, we risk misunderstanding and hindering their potential to develop positive connections with adults and the broader community. To engage adolescents, and to bridge the generational gap, we can start by accepting that they have a unique perspective. If we challenge our assumptions about adolescents and break out of our own memories and biased perspectives, we can forge more meaningful connections with the teens in our lives. When we are open to adolescents and their individual outlook instead of lecturing or insisting they conform, we will empower them to use their energy and innovation to repair our world.

●● Group Learning and Discussion ●●

This chapter reminds us of the complexity of the lives of youth. We cannot hope to influence their behavior if we do not understand the world they must navigate. There are no specific "practice" exercises in this section. Rather, the insights gained here should universally inform how we approach youth and how we propose they initiate positive behavioral changes in their lives.

There is a likelihood, however, that this chapter reminded you of the complexity of your own "adolescent world." This gives you an opportunity for self-reflection. When you understand your own adolescence, you are one step closer to understanding the adult you have become. You also may more readily note where you are "stuck"—to better comprehend why certain situations or people make you reactive or apprehensive. In particular, you may better grasp why certain adolescents you care for might trigger buttons within you that were installed long ago. When you are equipped with these insights, you are better prepared to serve youth.

■ References

1. Atwood M. *Cat's Eye*. New York, NY: Doubleday; 1988
2. Ginsburg KR; American Academy of Pediatrics Committee on Communications, Committee on Psychosocial Aspects of Child and Family Health. The importance of play in promoting healthy child development and maintaining strong parent-child bonds. *Pediatrics*. 2007;119(1):182–191
3. Corsaro WA. *The Sociology of Childhood*. Thousand Oaks, CA: Sage Publications; 1997
4. Reiner R. *Stand By Me* [videorecording]. Burbank, CA: RCA/Columbia Pictures Home Video
5. Savage D. It Gets Better Project. What is the It Gets Better Project? http://www.itgetsbetter.org/pages/about-it-gets-better-project. Accessed August 29, 2013

■ Related Video Content

2.0 The Adolescent World: Who Said Anything About the Teen Years Being Care Free? Youth.

2.1 The Adolescent World: Navigating School Pressures. Youth.

2.2 The Adolescent World: Navigating Relationships at Home. Youth.

2.3 The Adolescent World: Navigating a Stressful Environment. Youth.

2.4 The Adolescent World: Being Held to Low Expectations. Youth.

2.5 The Adolescent World: Building a Family When the One at Home May Have Let You Down. Youth.

2.6 The Adolescent World: Comfort With Diversity. Youth.

2.7 The Adolescent World: A Time of Fun and Discovery. Youth.

2.8 Thoughts on Parenting: The Voice of Adolescents. Youth.

3.5 Peers and Friendships: The Voice of Youth. Youth.

4.5 Teen-Produced Song: Paper Tigers. Youth, Toro.

10.9 Behaviors Must Be Seen in the Context of the Lives Youth Have Needed to Navigate. Auerswald.

CHAPTER 3

Friendships and Peers

Sara B. Kinsman, MD, PhD

 Related Video Content

3.0 Peers and Friendships: Insights Into the Complex Positive and Negative Impact Youth Have on Each Other

◼ Why This Matters?

When teens spend what can seem like an excessive amount of time talking, texting, skyping, and just simply hanging out with peers, it is important to remember that they are doing incredibly important developmental work. They are learning to manage conflict and get along with friends. To become a young adult capable of living, studying, and working with peers—independent from their parents—teens need to spend much of the second decade of their lives understanding who these people are and how to get along with them.

Parents and professionals equipped with a better understanding of peer culture and how to guide youth in navigating peer relationships will be positioned to support both safe behaviors and growing independence.

> **Peer relationships are the template for adult social, romantic, economic, and collegial relationships. In fact, peer interactions develop essential life skills connected to success, such as the ability to respond and grow from constructive criticism and develop leadership and collaborative strategies. For these reasons, it is important that we view youth separating from adults, adopting their own norms, and attending to their peers as a sign of appropriate developmental progress.**

◼ Appreciating Growing Independence and the Developmental Necessity of Peer Relationships

Most teens end up not too dissimilar from their parents, but rarely does a teen or young adult want to be exactly like their parent. Instead, teens create a unique generational subculture. Nevertheless, most teen subcultures to some degree do mimic the adult social life reflected in their families. In this way, teens can say, *"I am going to grow up, be an adult, but not exactly like my parents. I am independent."* If teens never developed a sense of separateness from their parents, they would be limited in taking care of themselves and ultimately in functioning as adults.

The need to attach to peers, however, is more than a stepping-stone toward independence from parents. It is a biological necessity that represents the first step toward romantic relationships and functioning as adults. Peer relationships are the template for adult social, romantic, economic, and collegial relationships. In fact, peer interactions develop essential life skills connected to success, such as the ability to respond and grow from constructive criticism and develop leadership and collaborative strategies. For these reasons, it is important that we view youth separating from adults, adopting their own norms, and attending to their peers as a sign of appropriate developmental progress. If, on the other hand, we deride peer cultures altogether, or become overly controlling in an effort to undermine peer relationships, adolescents will reflexively reject our views and actions as impeding their drive toward independence and self-sufficiency.

■ The Peer World

There are many layers of social complexity and many directions in which teens can influence one another.

Crowds

Studies over several decades have found that many adolescents self-identify with 1 of 4 general crowds: elites/populars, athletes/jocks, academics, and deviants.[1] A fifth group comprises those who fall outside the 4 main crowds or socialize between. Teens in this crowd have referred to themselves over time as "normals," "nobodies," "hybrids," "outcasts," or "loners," to name a few. The general tenor of the 4 major crowds has stayed consistent in US non-minority schools in the last few decades though the names of some crowds have changed over time. (Deviants have self-identified as "stoners," "druggies," "burnouts," "freaks," "punks," and "hoods.") Understanding crowd affiliation helps outsiders get a quick overview of how teens see themselves and their social world. When asked, teens may tell you how they do or do not fit into a crowd. This can be helpful, because you can start to understand the school culture the teen is dealing with and the benefits and pressures of fitting in, especially if a teen explains they have 2 sets of friends, the "skaters" and the "math geeks," for example.

Self-identified crowd affiliation may also tell us something about risk exposure. Brown and other's[1] findings suggest that students who say they were part of a deviant group were more likely to smoke cigarettes, use illicit drugs, and engage in nonconforming behaviors—perhaps, a way to join nonmainstream adult roles, including musicians, artists, or tradesmen. Students who were part of a popular group were more likely to use alcohol or have sex—perhaps taking on a lifestyle that mimics their ideas about college. Crowds are a general affiliation, and we must be aware to not over-stereotype. For example, the tattooed "deviant-looking" teen may be the leader of the math team.

Cliques

Because general associations do not tell us how individual teens make decisions, it can be helpful to understand the next layer of potential peer influence.[2] Cliques or smaller peer groups create subsets of teens who are more closely affiliated than crowds. Cliques can have a negative connotation because the peer group creates cohesion, in part, by separating themselves from or excluding others. For example, a group of 6 guys who are excellent football players (in the jock crowd) start elite training to ensure future scholarships, study hard, and avoid alcohol and all party-related activities. By creating a subset with unique norms, this clique within a crowd has a different set of health-risk issues (eg, becoming overly focused on nutrition and body fat) than their general crowd affiliation (eg, drinking alcohol).

Cliques typically have a hierarchy. One young student explained,

> Bob was at the top, number 1, and Max was number 2. They were pretty much the most popular people. Then there was a jump between them and the rest of the group. Nobody was at 3, but Marcus was a 3½, and so were 3 other guys. A few people were at 3¾, then Josh was a 4 and John was a 4. Everyone else moved between 3½ and 4, including me.[2]

Top-tier students generally maintain their rank, while lower-ranked students rarely ascend to the upper ranks. A good deal of research suggests that breaking into the top tier is very hard. The top tier comprises popular clique leaders who are well liked by their friends and almost serve as role models. It is not that these teens act like adults, but they definitely know how *not* to act like a child. These higher-status teens are more likely to look physically older; act a little older; be attractive; have excellent social skills; come from a high socioeconomic background; and actually initiate, or insinuate that they are initiating, slightly more mature behaviors.[3] For example, a 15-year-old may brag that she knows how to drive so well that, if she could, she would take her test today. She is certain that she would pass, and she is sure that her dad would be so impressed that he would let her drive everyone to the beach. None of this may be realistic, but the idea that she is thinking ahead and sounding so confident can make other teens in the group admire her and be a little envious simultaneously. For minority youth, maintaining status can be a bit more complex because they need to maintain their own cultural identity within a school structure that may differ in cultural values and perspectives.[4]

The clique represents a group that does not mind conforming to one another. Tightly conforming cliques peak during early adolescence, when there is a strong desire to conform. Eleven- to 13-year-olds are more apt to conform to perceived group opinions and are more likely to question themselves, not their peers, when confronted with a discrepancy.[5] This need to conform is usually not bearing down from the group leader or the other members of the clique. Rather, it is a teen's internal desire to avoid appearing different and risk not conforming. If you think about how a school of fish swims, 1 or 2 fish do not command the others to follow, rather the leaders and followers read one another well enough to stick together. Interestingly, not only does age affect how a teen will conform, but younger teens are more apt to conform to positive or pro-social behaviors and older teens are more apt to take risks. Older teens' desire to easily conform starts to wane as their tolerance for risk increases.[6] These studies suggest that pressure to conform is multidimensional. It varies by age, gender, direction of influence (positive and negative), type of behavior (pro-social and deviant), clique, and crowd affiliation.[5-8]

One of the tricky issues when we study peer pressure is deciding what behavior is deviant. When are teens following cues from peers and moving away from adult norms? Interestingly, peers spend a great deal of time talking, gossiping, and trying to figure out how to look like and become a young adult. Most times when a teen follows their peers, they are experimenting with behaviors that they assume will make them look older. The most likely behaviors that lend themselves to peer influence are age-inappropriate (eg, drinking alcohol and having sex) and not socially deviant (eg, stealing or physically harming others).[9] This is important, because most parents do not need to veer our teens away from risky peers, rather we need to be prepared that peers with slightly higher status will role-model or suggest age-inappropriate behaviors.[10,11]

If a teen does veer away from good friends to spend time with higher-risk peers, a caring adult needs to take a step back and wonder if there is a bigger problem. Teens who abruptly and completely redirected their friendships toward crowds and cliques that are not consistent with previous affiliations are struggling. This is not an expected part of adolescent social development. Without being critical of the new affiliations, a caring adult needs to understand why this change came about rather than berating the new peers.

Brea, a ninth grader who has always enjoyed spending time with friends from grade school and playing her flute, announces that she hates being in the band, is quitting, and finds her old friends stupid. She has started hanging out with kids who are known to skip school, smoke cigarettes, and dress provocatively. When you ask about the positives of spending time with her new friends, she explains, *"They are realistic about life. They know that almost everything in life is fake—just a show. They don't take any bullsh-t."* After you affirm that a "take no BS attitude" might be helpful in some situations, Brea agrees. She then tells you that she saw one of her parent's e-mail accounts and learned they are having an affair. They are repeatedly lying "to everybody" about having to go on "business trips," even missing her birthday.

Taking time to understand her dilemma, which was signaled by her change in friends, allowed a caring adult to step in and help her with this painful secret.

Maturity

Markers of maturity and independence are moving targets that are continually being reinterpreted. For example, a marker of increased independence at one age—cool blue Kool-Aid dyed hair—loses its currency and seems passé quickly. How peer groups message about continuously changing norms can be subtle. With gaze, gestures, stance, touch, teasing, chitchat, gossip, storytelling, and sometimes direct instruction (eg, how to French kiss or how to put on eyeliner), teens correct one another just enough to be creative, but not too far from the agreed-on norms of their clique's roadmap toward becoming an older version of themselves. Importantly, usually peer influence is very subtle, but sometimes the peer group can be overtly directive.

> In an 11th grade health class, students were asked to write down their private questions about sex and sexual health. The teacher read one card, *"Is there something wrong with you if you're a virgin at 16?"* As the question was read, the class boomed out of control. All the students, both boys and girls, were pointing and yelling to one another, *"Who is a virgin?"* Accusingly, they would point at different girls and said, *"Yeah, you're a virgin!"* The taunting continued, and the girls in question would respond, *"No, I'm no virgin!"*

This type of peer pressure dramatizes the power of peers to profoundly influence how a teen feels about her (or his) private decisions. In this school context, being a virgin was not the norm. In another school context, being a virgin could be the norm. What is interesting about moments of overt peer pressure is that we can all easily sympathize with how difficult it can feel to be the only one who is different. Of course, the teen who raised the question privately was not the only virgin, but the class response would lead each teen present to feel that they may be the only "deviant" teen in the class. These types of interactions are not typical in classrooms, but they are ever-present in more subtle dynamics. Their impact is best grasped when we understand they occur just as teens are hoping to pretty much look like everyone else, while keeping up with their peers, all while grappling with the internal desire to feel a bit more mature and a bit less like a child.

■ What Can Parents and Adults Do to Support Good, Healthy Friendships?

Professionals can play a pivotal role in supporting positive adolescent behaviors when they prepare them to manage the peer environment. However, our highest yield may be in guiding parents in how to prepare their children to navigate the world happily and safely.[12,13] Ideally, this preparation would happen early in childhood. Therefore, this section models how you might also discuss peers and friendships with parents of younger children. The talking points presented are divided among developmental ages, but should not be thought of as distinct. In fact, parents who have open communication and active involvement in the early years set the tone for ongoing deeper conversations during more advanced developmental stages.

The Early Years

- Starting from the preschool years, you can be present and available when your children are playing with others. You can provide instruction about sharing and resolving conflicts without hitting or demeaning friends. These early play times allow you to see how your child interacts with other children and highlights your child's internal social strengths and challenges. If your child is very shy, you will be able to help warm up initial interactions and, conversely, if your child is very social, you will be able to help him learn how to make room for a quieter friend.

- Even from the very start, children get very angry with friends. This gives you the opportunity to teach how to feel the emotional and physical sensation of anger and express anger without verbally or physically hurting others. It is also key to remember that anger is temporary. Your child needs to learn not to ruin a relationship out of momentary anger or frustration; the moment will pass.

The School-aged Years

- Adults often think "children need to work it out themselves." Sometimes they do. But rarely do people learn the fine art of friendship without some support or role-modeling about healthy friendships.

- Children with different social skills will require different coaching about friendships. The shy child will need to learn to not respond to peer conflict with fear, worry, and increased isolation. The child with attention-deficit/hyperactivity disorder will need to be coached to slow down or filter their thoughts so that they can give their friend "a break" before being too direct or harsh. A very physically active child will have to be sure to avoid hurting friends when filled with frustration and anger. Children who have grown up in a home where a lot of anger is expressed or children who have experienced or witnessed physical violence at home will need specific skills to slow down their physical and verbal response to a threat.

- Welcome your child's friends to your home. Be sure that they can follow the rules of your home. If speaking with respect and asking permission to have a snack is a core value in your family, be sure that your child's friends can accept and accommodate these rules. If a friend is difficult for you to manage, this will give you good information about what your child is coping with and whether you need to be involved in supporting or redirecting this friendship choice.

- If there is any chance that you can join your child's school, sport, or club event, get involved. Some preteens may ask that your involvement not "embarrass them," but still be present. In these settings, preteens may ignore you and almost forget you are there. You will get the chance to see your child in action and appreciate how they get along with their peers.

- Be sure that you, as a parent, are involved in creating social plans. There is no reason to encourage texting or phone use before a child needs it to keep in contact with you. Once she is able to remotely communicate with peers, be sure you know who she is communicating with, how much time she is in communication, and the nature of what she is communicating about. Devices should be put away when the family is hanging out (parents included).

- Though friends are important, emphasize early that so too is family time.

- Some children will identify a best friend. This can be very helpful, as the duo can take on new challenges and bounce ideas off one another. Knowing your child's best friend's family can be helpful. You can help your child decide when the friendship is supporting her to take on new developmental challenges and when one or the other child might feel burdened by being a best friend to the exclusion of others. Early best friends allow you to start the dialogue about the lifelong challenge of balancing time with close friends, groups of friends, and family.

- Remember that peer relationships are the most important relationships, beyond the family, to teach children empathy. You can help your child identify how she feels when a friendship creates a disappointment. You can help her identify her own emotions, such as feeling rejected, angry, hurt, or sad, and then pay attention to the larger social interaction. This can allow her to empathize with her friend rather than just feel her own emotion. Guide her to learn that she should act only after her own emotions have been identified and she has considered her friend's emotions or motives.

- Friendships offer the opportunity to learn about talking and listening. Children and adults need to learn that when you talk to a friend, that friend needs to be able just to listen. This is an ideal point to role-model.

- Parents can use friendships to drive home essential points about resilience. When a child chooses to talk to a friend about a concern, issue, or anything that made them upset, it is a sign they are a good friend. Figuring out how to communicate well with other people can be a significant source of strength.

- Teach that working things through with a friend is smart—you can avoid a fight (which usually only leads to more fighting anyway), save face because you took on (for boys, "manned up" to) the problem and, most importantly preserved meaningful friendships. Teaching children to preserve friendships with all their ups and downs is a tremendous skill that will bring lifelong stability in all personal relationships, including romantic ones.

- When a good friend moves away, this is a significant loss. But it also gives your child a chance to maintain a friendship over a distance. These friendships can provide a respite from school or sport friendships that have to deal with day-to-day hassles.

The Adolescent Years

- Many risks that teens take on are proxy markers of maturity—signals that teens send to others that they are ready to be seen as a young adult. This is when you worry about negative peer influences. It is true that most of the major health risks in life are started during adolescence and in the presence of peers—cigarette smoking, alcohol use, exposure to sexually transmitted infections, and possibly even obesity. It is understandable and important for you to have concerns about the potentially negative aspects of peer influence. However, it is also important for you to remember that peer influence can also be protective and peer support can be invaluable.

- Children at different ages require more support. First it is important to know when your child is most vulnerable. Younger adolescents are most apt to conform to perceived group opinions and more likely to question their own opinion than even younger children or older peers. Your child may pass through this stage at age 11 to 13 or 13 to 15, and some late bloomers will be more vulnerable later. Knowing how your child is maturing in relation to their peers is important.

- In middle school, friends and friendships can seem to change. A friend who always loved to play with dolls will decide that such play is immature and want to be on her iPad texting others. A group of guys who could play street soccer all day now opts to stay inside and just play video games.

- Know your child's "crowd" and understand how fitting into that crowd might create a "role" for them. For example, if your child is a popular student they may be a bit more adept socially than their peers, look or act a bit older, and can be influential. This can all be quite positive. But, they sometimes are aware that they have to try to act older than their peers to keep their popularity up. This can be a risk for them.

- As teens reach high school, friends get involved in different activities and friendship groups can become more diverse, but close friends might be better matched than in the earlier years. Some friends who have a new boyfriend or girlfriend will seem to just disappear.

- Teens develop social skills by hanging out with their peers. How to meet new people, converse in a group, make small talk, be teased and gently tease back, and generally share funny stories or jokes is one of the most important parts of friendship. Later in life, good friends will meet after a long break and often say it feels as comfortable to talk as when they first met in their teen or young adult years. In part, that is because they quickly get to the core of who the other person is, have a shared past, and often laugh at the same type of humor. Learning how to share your sense of humor with friends is critically important for social development because it can offset conflicts, mitigate criticism, and make life in general more fun.

- Encourage your teen to talk about all kinds of things with their peers. In conversations with peers, teens can have a back-and-forth discussion that feels more mutual than with adults who may have "already made up their mind" and inadvertently do not allow the teen to explore a range of ideas. Peers can be protective of your teen.

- Having a caring adult who is adept and "friended" without limits on your teen's social network page is important. It ensures that you "know" to some degree the feel, humor, and different types of people that your child connects with.

- Rather than blaming a teen who is vulnerable to peer pressure for "not being able to stand up" to others, it can be helpful to know that you will need to rely on "face-saving" strategies to help your child stay safe. This will better allow your child to be different from peers. Parents deciding that a preteen cannot go on a sleepover to a home with poor adult supervision makes the parent look like "a huge pain," but the preteen is spared potentially difficult decisions at the sleepover that he was not ready to face.

- One of the best things you can do to support good behaviors is to connect with the parents of your teen's friends. Remember that one of the fundamental questions for adolescents is, *"Am I normal?"* and sometimes they will make unwise decisions to prove they are normal. If they are given clearer or stricter boundaries than their friends, they may feel as if they are being treated unfairly and rebel as a result. On the other hand, when parents work together to create common expectations, your teens do not feel like they are being treated differently and will more comfortably comply with the rules.

◼ Teaching a Young Person Peer Navigation Skills[14]

A young person can be well informed, highly motivated to do the right thing, and poised to take action and still find herself unable to follow through on her intentions if she is not equipped with the skills that will enable her to implement her plans successfully.[15] The importance of possessing skills is a vital part of any behavioral change strategy. Without skills, any action is unlikely to meet with success, and the subsequent failure may generate frustration that will increase stress and may prevent a person from trying again.[16] Skills are essential to creating the genuine sense of competence that gives a person well-earned confidence. The skills needed to promote safe behaviors range from properly using a bike helmet or seat belt to correctly using a condom. The discussion here, however, will focus on the skills youth need to successfully navigate the pressures and influences of their peers.[17] These skills can be broken into 3 categories. ▶ 3.1

1. Learning to say no
2. Recognizing manipulation and successfully navigating around it
3. Shifting the blame to save face

These skills may be ideally taught in the presence of parents because they can reinforce the lessons and are actually integral parts of the plan for adolescents. You can directly teach the skills in an office visit or raise the subject and distribute the supplemental materials.

Learning to Say "No!"

When the word "no" is used equivocally, it leads to conflicting double messages, particularly in sexual circumstances. When "no" is said with a smile or giggle, it is interpreted as "keep asking." These mixed signals can lead to continual pressure or even date rape. Too often, adolescents explain that they don't like to say no because "it sounds mean." You are not asking them to be mean, just to be clear. In fact, suggest that, when they mean yes, they should also just say "yes" and then take steps to ensure they are safe.

Teens need to learn to say no in a clear, firm tone and make it nonnegotiable. Even consider practicing this vital skill with youth in your office. Be prepared that this may be somewhat embarrassing, and they may do so with a smile. This gives you an opportunity to point out how a smile coupled with the word "no" conveys a confusing message.

In preparing parents for adolescence, we can guide parents of younger children to use the word "no" rarely, and to reserve it for only when they mean it. Many children learn early in life that, if they continue to ask, they can turn their parents' initial denial into a "well, maybe," and finally a "yes." Learning that "no means no" in their early years can make it easier for preteens and teens to understand that message clearly when they have to say no themselves. Parents should feel comfortable saying "maybe" or "I'll have to consider it," instead of a reflexive "no" when they may just be tired or don't really mean no.

Recognizing Manipulation and Successfully Navigating Around It

Peer pressure is usually subtle. Often, words are not even exchanged. Rather, it is internally driven: *"If I do this, I'll fit in."* or *"If I do it just once, I'll earn my way into the popular crowd."* or *"He really will love me if I just let him."* Although most peer pressure is internally driven, young people still do receive pressure-filled, manipulative messages from peers.

A commonly taught way to prepare young people to deal with manipulation is to teach them to recognize a line and then to respond by reversing the pressure. For example, *"Let's get drunk. I'll bet you'll be a funny drunk. You're my best friend and everybody else is already doing it every weekend,"* would elicit a response like, *"Well, I'm not like everybody else, and I don't need to drink with you to be your friend."* This strategy ignores how much teens are driven to be accepted. While they may understand how to implement this technique, they may not actually use it if it puts them in conflict with their friends.

A slightly modified way to handle this kind of pressure allows adolescents not to have to challenge their friends while still controlling their own actions. The technique has 3 stages.

1. They need to be able to recognize a line. Parents can reinforce this skill using commercial manipulation as a teaching tool or while watching television. You can also suggest they do it while driving around and witnessing teen behaviors. The key to minimizing resistance is to keep the discussion away from situations that are personal to the teen.
2. They need to be taught how to firmly state their positions with no ambivalence without being argumentative, accusatory, or condescending. *"I'm not getting drunk." "I'm not ready for sex." "I'm not cheating."*
3. They offer an alternative that allows them to continue the relationship on their terms but doesn't challenge the friendship. *"I won't get drunk, but if you can still stand up, I'll shoot hoops with you later." "I love you, too, but I'm not ready for sex. I still want to be with you and we can have fun, even feel good, in other ways." "I'm not bad at biology, so if you want, I'll get you caught up."*

Shifting the Blame to Save Face

Adolescents are better equipped to deal with peer pressure and other negative influences if they can get out of difficult situations without losing face or compromising standing with peers. Teens may know the rational decision to make, but if that choice doesn't play well in peer culture, they may choose not to follow their own common sense.[18] The following 2 techniques are designed to offer adolescents a way out while still fitting in, essentially by shifting blame to their parents.

The Check-in Rule

The check-in rule is a logical extension of parental monitoring. It is a bedtime routine not unlike the one families may have with younger children. While it is unusual for a younger child to get to bed without some parental involvement—a story, a bath, prayer, or help with homework—adolescents often go to bed without such a routine. They are sometimes allowed to arrive home after parents have themselves gone to sleep.

The check-in rule has to be used every time, no exceptions. No matter what time the adolescent arrives home, she must say goodnight to her parent(s), even if it means awakening them. This creates opportunities for some very important discussions. Having a nightly "check-in rule" also helps adolescents shift blame to parents. Teens have a face-saving reason to avoid drinking or staying out too late: *"Are you kidding? My mom smells me!"* This strategy of parental monitoring allows a teen to better maintain self-control. The teen also may be more likely to do the right thing just because he knows his parents care enough to be paying attention.

Code Words

With this technique, the parent and adolescent choose a code word or phrase not to be shared with friends and to be used only in an emergency. "Emergency" is defined as any situation in which the adolescent needs to leave a risky social situation and feels uncomfortable or at risk for not being able to get out safely on his own. He calls or texts home in front of his friends, ideally so they can clearly hear or view his end of the conversation. He informs his parents that he will be out late or tells them where he will be going, presumably to ask permission. He casually inserts the code, perhaps *"Yeah, I won't be home so I can't walk Sparky."* Sparky is their agreed-on code word. When the father hears it, he knows his son is in a difficult situation, so he raises his voice loud enough for the friends to overhear and demands his son comes home. If the son can get home safely, he leaves, all the while complaining about his overbearing father. If he can't get home on his own, he rejects his father's instructions to return home, prompting his father to demand he meet him outside in 5 minutes. The code word works best when it comes with an agreement that teens will not be punished for reaching out for help, even if they were involved in something parents would not approve of.

A code word is an ideal addition to the "Contract for Life" promoted by Students Against Destructive Decisions.[19] In that contract, the teen promises to call home for a ride if there is any reason to believe driving may not be safe, particularly if the driver has been using substances. In turn, the parent(s) agrees to provide a safe ride without an accompanying punishment. The contract assumes the teen will have the ability to call parents from within a social, peer-charged context. If a code word is added to the contract, it may make it easier for the teen to place that call or text home.

●● Group Learning and Discussion ●●

Break into pairs. First, practice having a conversation with parents about their important role in supporting healthy friendships. Then, practice guiding teens on how to navigate peer culture safely by discussing the key communication skills and negotiation skills discussed in this chapter. Finally, hold a discussion with parents on the check-in rule and implementing a code word as firm family safety rules.

■ References

1. Sussman S, Pokhrel P, Ashmore RD, Brown BB. Adolescent peer group identification and characteristics: a review of the literature. *Addict Behav.* 2007;32(8):1602–1627
2. Adler PA, Adler P. *Peer Power: Preadolescent Culture and Identity.* Piscataway, NJ: Rutgers University Press; 1998
3. Coleman JS. *The Adolescent Society: The Social Life of the Teenager and Its Impact on Education.* Oxford, England: Free Press of Glencoe; 1961
4. Fordham S, Ogbu J. Black students' school success: coping with the "burden of acting white." *Urban Rev.* 1986;18(3):176–206
5. Costanzo PR, Shaw ME. Conformity as a function of age level. *Child Dev.* 1966;37(4):967–975
6. Berndt T. Developmental changes in conformity to peers and parents. *Dev Psychol.* 1979;15(6):608–616
7. Brown BB, Lohr MJ, McClenahan E. Early adolescents' perceptions of peer pressure. *J Early Adolesc.* 1986;6(2):139–154
8. Clasen DR, Brown BB. The multidimensionality of peer pressure in adolescence. *J Youth Adolesc.* 1985;14(6):451–468
9. Kinsman SB, Romer D, Furstenberg FF, Schwarz DF. Early sexual initiation: the role of peer norms. *Pediatrics.* 1998;102(5):1185–1192
10. Snyder J, Dishion TJ, Patterson GR. Determinants and consequences of associating with deviant peers during preadolescence and adolescence. *J Early Adolesc.* 1986;6(1):29–43
11. Dolcini MM, Adler NE. Perceived competencies, peer group affiliation, and risk behavior among early adolescents. *Health Psychol.* 1994;13(6):496–506
12. Romer D, Black M, Ricardo I, Feigelman S. Social influences on the sexual behavior of youth at risk for HIV exposure. *Am J Public Health.* 1994;84(6):977–985
13. Fletcher AC, Darling, NE, Steinberg L. The company they keep: relation of adolescents' adjustment and behavior to their friends' perceptions of authoritative parenting in the social network. *Dev Psychol.* 1995;31(2):300–310
14. Ginsburg KR, Jablow MM. *Building Resilience in Children and Teens: Giving Kids Roots and Wings.* 2nd ed. Elk Grove Village, IL: American Academy of Pediatrics; 2011
15. Prochaska JO, DiClemente CC. Stages of change in the modification of problem behaviors. *Prog Behav Modif.* 1992;28:183–218
16. Bandura A. *Social Learning Theory.* Englewood Cliffs, NJ: Prentice Hall; 1977
17. Velicer WF, Prochaska JO, Fava JL, et al. Smoking cessation and stress management: applications of the transtheoretical model of behavior change. *Homeostasis.* 1998;38:216–233
18. Gardner M, Steinberg L. Peer influence on risk taking, risk preference, and risky decision making in adolescence and adulthood: an experimental study. *Dev Psychol.* 2005;41(4):625–635
19. SADD Contract for Life. SADD, Inc., 2005. http://www.sadd.org/contract.htm. Accessed August 29, 2013

■ Related Video Content ▶

3.0 Peers and Friendships: Insights Into the Complex Positive and Negative Impact Youth Have on Each Other. Kinsman.

3.1 Peer Negotiation Strategies: Empowering Teens AND Parents. Ginsburg.

3.2 Media as a Super-peer. Rich.

3.3 Peer Relationships Can Tell Us so Much if We Don't Interrupt Disclosure With Judgment. Pletcher.

3.4 Peers, Partners, Friends, and Even Partners of Friends: Widening Circles of Influence. Diaz.

3.5 Peers and Friendships: The Voice of Youth. Youth.

3.6 Case Example: Guiding a Parent and Teen to Work Together to Address Substance Use. Sugerman.

3.7 Helping Youth With Chronic Illness Navigate Peer Relationships. Pletcher.

■ Related Handouts/Supplementary Materials

Doing the Right Thing...and Still Keeping Your Friends

Saying "NO!"...When You Really Mean It

Effective Monitoring: Joining with other Parents to Set Common Rules

■ Related Web Sites

Friends Are Important: Tips for Parents

www.healthychildren.org/FriendsAreImportant

This brochure ties in with the *Connected Kids* theme of the benefits of positive communication with your child about the benefits of friendships.

Connected Kids

www.aap.org/connectedkids

This is one practical approach for pediatricians to provide anticipatory guidance protocols such as Bright Futures and Guidelines for Health Supervision. The approach focuses positive friendships, anger management as a way of emphasizing the important of violence prevention.

KidsHealth: Helping Kids Cope With Cliques

http://kidshealth.org/parent/positive/talk/cliques.html

CHAPTER 4

Perfectionism

Kenneth R. Ginsburg, MD, MS Ed, FAAP, FSAHM
Susan T. Sugerman, MD, MPH, FAAP

 Related Video Content

4.0 Perfectionism: A Barrier to Authentic Success

■ Why This Matters?

We prepare youth to be successful when they are poised to be high achievers rather than perfectionists. Perfectionists feel unacceptable unless they produce a flawless product or performance.[1] Perfectionism is associated with a host of problems in adolescents, including eating disorders,[2-4] obsessive compulsive disorder (OCD),[5,6] depression and anxiety,[7,8] somatic symptoms,[7] and suicidality.[9]

The literature discusses adaptive and maladaptive perfectionism with the understanding that some degree of the drive toward being perfect may actually be good.[10] Here, a person with adaptive perfectionism will be termed a "healthy high achiever" and the maladaptive perfectionist will be referred to as a "perfectionist."

> **Teach parents how to support "healthy achievement" while minimizing the drive to maladaptive perfectionism, which may prevent outside-of-the box thinking and limit creative and innovative potential. Help parents teach their children to use mistakes and failures as learning opportunities for growth that generate long-term character and values and more genuine lifelong success.**

Perfectionists don't enjoy the creative process because their fear of failure is greater than the joy of experiencing success. They see mistakes as proof that they're unworthy. They are suspicious of others' praise because they view themselves as "imposters" whose faults remain undiscovered. They may experience constructive criticism as reinforcement of their inadequacy. Perhaps most limiting to future success, the thought of not doing something well may prevent them from thinking outside of the box, limiting their creative and innovative potential.

In contrast, healthy high achievers aren't satisfied until they've done their best and prove resilient when they fall short of perfection. Healthy high achievers enjoy the process and excitement as they work their hardest. They see mistakes as opportunities for growth and failures as temporary setbacks. They value constructive criticism as informative. They look for creative solutions and are willing to take healthy risks.

Not all perfectionists are high performers. Fear of failure may cause them to avoid a task entirely. Sometimes they project an image to make the pressure stop. Being perceived as "lazy" or even as a drug user can be viewed positively by some teens, whereas being anxious is not. The pressure of being perfect makes them go out of their way to build a strong case for indifference. This possibility should be considered when young people have a sudden drop in performance. These youth often receive negative feedback from home and may need professional guidance to be able to say, *"I act like I don't care because I care too much."*

■ What Factors Create Perfectionism?

There may be a biological component to perfectionism as evidenced by its link to eating disorders[2–4] and OCD.[5,6] Here we will focus on those environmental factors that may contribute to or exacerbate perfectionism.

Inappropriate Praise

Carol Dweck and colleagues[11] study the effect that praise and criticism have on performance and write about a "growth mindset" compared to a "fixed mindset." Young people with a growth mindset believe their intelligence can be developed with effort. When they do not produce desired results, they don't see themselves as failures, but as learners. People with a growth mindset want feedback because they understand they need others' assessments to learn to do things better. Dweck writes, *"The passion for stretching yourself and sticking to it, even (or especially) when it's not going well, is the hallmark of the growth mindset."*

In contrast, people with a fixed mindset (including maladaptive perfectionists and others) believe people are either smart or not and failure proves you're not. In fact, hard work suggests one doesn't have natural intelligence. Their goal becomes to avoid failure at all costs since they need consistent feedback to affirm they're smart. Dweck explains that people with a fixed mindset view situations from the prism of, *"Will I succeed or fail?" "Will I look smart or dumb?" "Will I win or lose?"* People with a growth mindset feel successful when they can do something they couldn't do before, whereas those with fixed mindsets feel smart when they avoid errors.

Dweck's research reveals that how a child is praised contributes heavily to whether she develops a growth versus fixed mindset. In brief, those praised for being smart are more likely to grow to fear being seen as anything else, and those noticed for effort develop a passion for growth.

Academic Pressures and a Competitive College Admissions Process

Parents and children alike see getting a college degree as important for long-term success and financial security. This often translates into external and internal pressure not simply to attain high grades and test scores, but also to build extensive resumes filled with impressive extra-curricular achievements. The competition is not limited to those applying to elite universities. Increases in the perceived importance of secondary education across society as well as the rising costs of tuition lead to anxiety among all students about competition for admission and scholarship dollars, especially in the context of difficult economic times.

Sensationalism of Success and Failure (ie, Who Are Our Heroes?)

Our culture reveres success and ridicules failure. The heroes in our society tend to epitomize a perfect performance in their fields and are rewarded with the greatest external trappings of success. Whether the highest-scoring athlete, the top-grossing recording artist, or the most beautiful movie actress, our sports stars and entertainment figures receive enormous attention, especially when at the "top of their game." When they have a transgression, the media quickly focuses on their problems. Youth receive the message that, to gain recognition, you must be at the top, and, once there, you had better not make a mistake.

Increase in a Permissive Style of Parenting

Permissive parents are very warm and supportive to their children but offer few boundaries or rules, often taking on a tone of "friendship" more than mentorship in their approach to parenting. The result is that teens' behavioral control is achieved largely through their desire to please parents. Achieving perfection can ensure the child pleases his parents, especially if the definition of what counts as "acceptable" is not clear.

Fear of Disappointment

Many perfectionists have a strong desire to avoid disappointing their parents, especially when raised in a permissive parenting style as noted above. Others are driven by the fear of disappointing themselves. Children who see themselves as valuable only when achieving success may experience significant cognitive dissonance when trying to accept a failure or limitation in performance or abilities. As a result, they pursue perfectionism as a means to avoid disappointment at all costs.

Applying Professional Standards to Personal Parenting

Some parents highly prepared for the work world apply the same standards of efficiency, productivity, and performance to family life. When this happens, their children's perceived successes or setbacks become markers of the parents' own success. This may intensify stress on children either directly through parental pressure or through their own drive to please adults.

Desire to Spare Stressed Parents

Teens sometimes have an intense need to spare a parent whom they perceive as stressed. Children whose parents suffer from trauma, illness, or divorce may try to be perfect children. They may keep their own anxieties and struggles as tightly held secrets, always showing parents their best face. Parents who explicitly verbalize feelings of being overwhelmed to their children or who excessively rely on their children as confidants about adult problems could exacerbate this.

■ Solutions

The professional can have 3 major roles in serving the adolescent with perfectionist tendencies: (1) assess for comorbid conditions (eg, anxiety, OCD) that may benefit from appropriate referral and treatment, (2) offer parents guidance on how to prevent or minimize perfectionism, (3) help youth who "have gotten off the playing field" and are perceived as being "lazy" to address their fear of failure. This can be healing for families because anger and disappointment can transform to more appropriate support.

Parents may or may not be one of the sources of perfectionism, but they certainly can be part of the solution. The above points present the areas you can use as topics of discussion. It is important in these discussions to remember that even parents who put a lot of pressure on their children do so with their children's best interest in mind. They should be gently guided to understand perfectionism not only feels uncomfortable but also interferes with success; the fear of failure associated with the need to be perfect can stifle creative and innovative thought and generate discomfort with constructive criticism. Following are a few topics you may want to draw from in your discussion with parents.

Effective Praise and Criticism

It is important that parents learn to praise effort rather than product. The statement, *"Just try your best,"* may be misunderstood by people with a high degree of internalized pressure. Those who have been capable of high performance or perfect scores in the past may take this to mean they should meet that standard on every task in the future. Instead, keep feedback and encouragement targeted. Explain that someone can try really hard yet perform quite differently in different subjects due to uneven strengths. **4.2**

- For example, instead of parents saying, *"Don't worry, I just expect you to do your best,"* say something like, *"All I expect is for you to put in a good effort. I care less about your grades and more about the fact that you are learning. Some things come easily to me, and with even a little effort I will always do well—for you, that's math. In other subjects, I might work really hard and still not do as well as I wish I could. But, all I want from you is to stretch yourself and learn; it's not the grades that matter. I know writing is hard for you, I'm proud when I see you keep working on it."*

- Teach parents to guide teens through self-evaluation based on the process rather than the outcome. They can ask, *"Do you think you spent a reasonable amount of time working on the project (or studying for the test)?" "Do you feel you learned what you needed to?" "Is there something you wish you did differently that you can change the next time?"* When youth learn from their own "imperfect" experiences without internalizing negativity, they can make real and meaningful changes to improve the process (and possibly outcome) in the future.

- Provide perspective about the costs of perfectionism (ie, just because you can doesn't always mean you should).

Most parents intuitively recognize the need for balance in managing the tasks of daily life. They can help their children work toward the same goal by teaching that perfectionism comes with costs to emotional and physical health. Time and energy are limited resources; one cannot sleep and study simultaneously. Extra time spent on a project may mean less time connecting with friends or doing a rewarding extracurricular activity. Parents may have to advocate for their children's need to get enough sleep, even when homework is not finished. Parents seeing their children suffer symptoms of exhaustion, isolation, anxiety, or depression may need to set limits on numbers of advanced classes taken or the degree of participation in outside activities.

Model Self-acceptance

Help parents present a "human" face to their children. Explain that children learn to internalize humility and self-respect when they see a parent admit and correct a mistake or failing, while witnessing parental self-deprecation for less than perfect achievement or talent sets children up to accept nothing less from themselves. Encourage parents to acknowledge their own limitations while celebrating their strengths, and hopefully their children will do the same.

Making Realistic Heroes

Talk to parents about the importance of discussing the real heroes all around us—those who choose to teach and to heal, those who choose to protect us and to serve our communities and nation. Encourage parents to talk about the acts of kindness they witness among neighbors. When children see realistic heroes and hear positive messages about the actions of real, accessible people, they learn a broader definition of success within which they, too, can feel valued.

Parents Need to Communicate That They Are Not Spared When Adolescents Keep Their Feelings Inside

You might consider discussing with parents whether their children notice their level of stress. As always, encourage parents that one of the best things they can do for their children's emotional well-being is to take care of themselves—to "put on their own oxygen mask first."

- Consider encouraging them to explain that, although they might be burdened, their greatest pleasure and most important job remains to parent them. You may consider encouraging them to say something like, *"I know you want to protect me from more worries, and I appreciate how much you care about me. But, the one thing I want to do right now more than anything is to be your mom/dad. Please let me to do that; I want to always be there for you."*

Encourage Parents to Be Clear About Their Definition of Success

Children absorb the definition of success from the media and broader culture. Some of those messages do not sit well with parents. Encourage parents to clarify and communicate their own views of success. You can't tell parents what those should be, but you might suggest some worthy contenders.

- Happiness, contentment
- Commitment to hard work, tenacity
- Resilience
- Generosity ✓
- Compassion and empathy ✓
- Desire to contribute
- Capacity to build and maintain meaningful relationships ✓
- Collaborative skills ✓
- Creativity and innovative potential
- Capacity to accept and learn from constructive criticism

Encourage Parents to Give Kids Opportunities for Self-discovery

Many parents assume that more is better—extra activities will build their resume. Enrichment activities are good, but we need to also encourage child-driven play and some down time.[12] To parents who would never let their kid be a "quitter," reframe it as "pruning." When kids feel overwhelmed, they can't focus on anything or learn where they excel. When they can prune away what no longer interests them, their strongest interests and greatest talents will flourish.

Unconditional Acceptance

If perfectionism is a state of discomfort driven by a fear of being unacceptable, the greatest antidote is unconditional acceptance. Parents need to consistently reinforce that their teens are acceptable just as they are.

You can reinforce that the most essential ingredient in raising resilient children is the connection parents form when they love or accept their children unconditionally and hold them to high but reasonable expectations. "High expectations" does not refer to grades or performance. It refers to their expectations for effort and of integrity, generosity, empathy, and other core values. Remind parents not to compare their adolescents to siblings or neighbors, because such comparisons impede feeling fully acceptable. Finally, although parents don't intend to imply conditional acceptance when they overfocus on grades and scores, children can misinterpret this attention as, *"If I bring home better grades, you'll love me more."*

Seeking Professional Help

Perfectionists may be so anxious and uncomfortable that they deserve professional help. First, the school should know how anxious the student is so that parents and the school together can convey supportive messages that reduce external pressures. However, sometimes a teen's perfectionism is internally driven by unhealthy thought patterns that reinforce what they "must" or "should" do lest their actions lead to catastrophic outcomes (eg, *"If I don't get an A, I will never get into college, I will never be able to become a doctor, and I will lose the love of my parents."*) In these cases, consider referral to a mental health specialist who includes cognitive behavioral therapy in treatment plans.

●● Group Learning and Discussion ●●

There are several key challenges in discussing perfectionism with adolescents and their families. The first is to do so without making the parent feel guilty or responsible; the key here is to emphasize that perfectionism comes from multiple sources and they may or may not be part of the problem, but they are certainly part of the solution. Second, it is important to help anxious parents understand that your goal is not to help their child achieve mediocrity; to the contrast it is to position him for authentic success. The third is to help parents understand that their "lazy" child may in fact care too much and may be masking his discomfort. In parallel, you hope to help the young person to be able to express that he is not lazy, it is just that he cares too much. Finally, it is your role to assess whether a higher level of care is needed, such as cognitive behavioral therapy, or even medication, in the case of anxiety or OCD.

Discuss in a group how perfectionism manifests among the teens you serve. Then break into pairs and work through the following cases.

Case 1: A 15-year-old girl is the daughter of immigrant parents. They have told her that the only way to make it in America is through an education. She has been told that there are no A minuses in their family. She studies until 1:00 to 2:00 every morning, taking breaks only for her violin lessons. She has daily abdominal pain, but has been told she is constipated. She loves her parents very much. They work 16- to 18-hour days so that she and her 2 siblings can go to the very best college. She doesn't want to disappoint them.

Case 2: A college professor brings in her 17-year-old son. His father is on international travel closing a business deal. He used to do quite well in school until he began changing. Now he has long blue hair and acts like he doesn't care at all about school. He is getting Cs and Ds except for in English class, where he loves talking about the innuendos hidden throughout the works of Shakespeare and Chaucer. He says his English teacher is cool, but the rest of school is lame.

Case 3: A distraught couple brings in their 13-year-old daughter. She studies all the time, sleeps little, and does not seem to be social. She worries incessantly that she is going to fail out of school, but what she means is that she might not get a 100 on her tests. Her parents insist that they just want her to be happy. They feel terrible that they used to tell her to study harder last year when she spent so much time at the mall with her friends. In a private interview, the girl tells you that she just knows her teachers will hate her if she fails out. She also knows that she'll never get to be a doctor if she fails now. To make sure that she does well, she spends a lot of time staying organized. All of her schoolwork and books are color-coded and in alphabetical order. She also worries about getting sick because she can't afford to miss school. To stay healthy, she keeps her room spotless and washes her hands repeatedly to make sure they are germ-free.

References

1. Greenspon TS. *Freeing Our Families From Perfectionism*. Minneapolis, MN: Free Spirit Publishing; 2002
2. Kirsh G, McVey G, Tweed S, Katzman DK. Psychosocial profiles of young adolescent females seeking treatment for an eating disorder. *J Adolesc Health*. 2007;40(4):351–356
3. Castro J, Gila A, Gual P, et al. Perfectionism dimensions in children and adolescents with anorexia nervosa. *J Adolesc Health*. 2004;35(5):392–398
4. Soenens B, Vansteenkiste M, Vandereycken W, Luyten P, Sierens E, Goossens L. Perceived parental psychological control and eating-disordered symptoms: maladaptive perfectionism as a possible intervening variable. *J Nerv Ment Dis*. 2008;196(2):144–152
5. Libby S, Reynolds S, Derisley J, Clark S. Cognitive appraisals in young people with obsessive-compulsive disorder. *J Child Psychol Psychiatry*. 2004;45(6):1076–1084
6. Ye HJ, Rice KG, Storch EA. Perfectionism and peer relations among children with obsessive-compulsive disorder. *Child Psychiatry Hum Dev*. 2008;39:415–426
7. Stoeber J, Rambow A. Perfectionism in adolescent school students: relations with motivation, achievement, and well-being. *Pers Individ Dif*. 2007;42(7):1379–1389
8. Hewitt PL, Carmen F, Caelian CF, et al. Perfectionism in children: associations with depression, anxiety, and anger. *Pers Individ Dif*. 2002;32(6):1049–1061
9. O'Connor RC. The relations between perfectionism and suicidality: a systematic review. *Suicide Life Threat Behav*. 2007;37(6):698–714
10. Enns MW, Cox BJ. The nature and assessment of perfectionism: a critical analysis. In: Flett GL, Hewitt PL, eds. *Perfectionism: Theory, Research and Treatment*. Washington, DC: American Psychological Association; 2002: 33–63
11. Dweck C. *Mindset: The New Psychology of Success*. New York, NY: Ballantine Books; 2006
12. Ginsburg KR; American Academy of Pediatrics Committee on Communications, Committee on Psychosocial Aspects of Child and Family Health. The importance of play in promoting healthy child development and maintaining strong parent-child bonds. *Pediatrics*. 2007;119(1);182–191

Related Video Content

4.0 Perfectionism: A Barrier to Authentic Success. Ginsburg.

4.1 Raising Children Prepared for Authentic Success. Ginsburg.

4.2 Using Praise Appropriately: The Key to Raising Children With a Growth Mind-set. Ginsburg.

4.3 We Must Not Assume "Perfect" Youth Are Problem-Free: They Need Us to Hear Their Struggles and Assess Their Behaviors. Campbell.

4.4 Because We Need to Learn How to Recover From Failure, Adolescence Needs to Be a Safe Time to Make Mistakes. Ginsburg.

4.5 Teen-Produced Song: Paper Tigers. Youth, Toro.

4.6 Managing School-Related Anxiety. Ginsburg.

4.7 Children of Divorce Can Become Perfectionists to Spare Their Parents. Sonis, Ginsburg.

4.8 Addressing Perfectionism in Military Youth. Youth, Lemmon, Ginsburg.

Related Handouts/Supplementary Materials

Don't Spare Me! Help Your Child Understand that You Want to Be There When They Need You, Even if You are Busy or Stressed

Helping Your Child…be a High Achiever instead of a Perfectionist

CHAPTER 5

Grief

Alison Culyba, MD, MPH
Sara B. Kinsman, MD, PhD

 Related Video Content

5.0 Supporting Youth Through the Grieving Process

■ Why This Matters

Grief is a universal experience. Approximately 2 million children and adolescents in the United States have experienced a parental death. Half of all marriages end with divorce, creating family conflict for countless teens. Neighborhoods are gripped by violence, with teens losing family and friends unexpectedly. Caregivers suffer from chronic physical and mental illnesses that render them unable to fully participate in family life. Loved ones are deployed for extended periods to serve our nation. All of the youth we care for will experience grief at some point. Helping adolescents effectively cope with loss builds resilience and allows them to develop a coping skill set that they can carry forth into adulthood.

> Grieving adolescents learn an essential life skill—how to survive loss. As they grieve, they develop a deeper understanding of their emotions. They come to understand their profound capacity for love. And they ultimately find that, despite the depth of sadness, they are able to heal and again find joy.

■ Grappling With Loss

Grief can emerge for adolescents through the loss of a parent, a sibling, a grandparent, or a very good friend, or loss of an animal that is considered part of the family. Grief can also occur due to serious medical or mental illness in the family that renders someone unable to connect in a meaningful way. When families are separated by divorce or military deployment, adolescents can also experience grief at the change in family structure. Some losses, such as those experienced when family members suffer from terminal illness, are prolonged. Others are sudden and unexpected, such as the loss of a friend to gun violence. Violent deaths can cause severe stress responses as well as a strong desire to seek revenge. Both foreseeable and unexpected losses can bring with them profound grief. Understanding the depth of the loss requires insight into the individual relationship between the adolescent and their deceased family member or friend.

Adolescence is a particularly challenging time to grapple with grief and loss. Teens attempt to seek out meaningful and lasting relationships with both adults and peers. They begin to form unique relationships, with each relationship providing them with a special kind of connection. When one of these relationships ends abruptly, it can be particularly jarring. Further, in contrast to younger children, adolescents have a more complete understanding of the permanence of death.

Losing a loved one is a physically painful process. It can be all-consuming and over-whelming. For many, the adolescent years will be the first time they experience these intense emotions. They may be surprised by the depth and intensity of emotions they feel in response to the loss. They often feel as though their world has come to a stop. Yet they see the busy world around them continuing to carry on while they struggle with intense sadness. You may hear adolescents say things like, *"How can these people be out getting coffee when my grandmother just died?"* or *"How are they laughing?"* They grapple with how to fill the void left by the person who passed on.

■ Loss Affects Family Functioning

Loss becomes more complicated because it affects the way an entire family functions. When the loss involves a member of the nuclear family, it usually causes the family to function poorly. Suddenly, family roles can change. An adolescent who thought of her mom as the family foundation becomes confused when she sees that her mom cannot cope with her father's death. As parents deal with their own grief, they may become less available to their children and cease to function as leaders of the family. People around them may say things like, *"You just lost your grandmother, but your mom is here."* or *"You are so lucky to have such a great dad to help you through this."* However, in reality, the mom or dad may not be functioning well in their parenting role following a loss. Teens are very perceptive regarding these role changes. They may feel abandoned. The sense of, *"Oh no, who is tak-ing care of me?"* can be very real.

■ Making Sense of a Loss

Teens can react in many ways to loss. Teens (and adults suffering a loss of someone they are very connected to) may continue to experience a loved one's presence. Sometimes you will learn that the teen continues to sense the presence of the person they lost and will even feel comforted talking with that presence. Adolescents may say, *"My mom is always with me. I feel she is always there."* or *"My grandmother talks to me while I am sleeping."*

Other teens will experience comfort in the smell or feel of their loved one. Younger adolescents often seek out physical items such as clothing and accessories that belonged to the lost loved one in order to further solidify this bond. These are helpful ways for adolescents to cope with the loss and transition from having their loved one close by.

■ Common Adolescent Behavior Changes

Adolescence is a developmentally complicated period in which individuals are exploring their own self-identity and defining their relationships. They are seeking more indepen-dence. They are also moving from very concrete to more abstract thought processes. These developmental changes can be challenging under the best of circumstances. However, in times of stress, these processes become even more challenging.

It is important to keep these developmental changes in mind when thinking about normal adolescent responses to grief. In some ways, adolescents deal with grief similarly to adults. The adult classic model of the stages of grief first described by Dr Elisabeth Kubler-Ross in 1969 (denial, anger, bargaining, depression, and acceptance) applies to some degree to adolescents. However, it is essential to explore adolescents' grief responses within a developmental framework in order to understand the deeper driving forces. While adolescent development occurs on a continuum, it is helpful to explore the distinct responses of early and late adolescents.

Early adolescence (about ages 12–14) is a particularly challenging time to experience loss. During this time, adolescents are working to withdraw emotionally from parents in order to gain more independence and gain peer acceptance. There is often tremendous internal conflict between wanting to be dependent versus independent. Early adolescents' grief frequently manifests as anger as they struggle with these 2 forces. They may wish to avoid all emotional expression, especially any public display of emotion. They can become angry or dismissive if an adult begins to cry in front of others. They may allow their emotions to come out in private, often crying alone in their rooms. This can create tension within a family because older adults feel the teen pulling away just in a moment when most adults seek closeness. And while early adolescents want to spend more time with friends, they are extremely apprehensive about confiding in friends for fear of being rejected by their peer group.

Some younger adolescents tend to become busy with their school and extracurricular activities following the loss of a loved one. Boys in particular respond to grieving this way. They may immediately want to go back to school. They fill their days with schoolwork, games, and activities. This offers a distraction from the all-encompassing grieving that is typically going on at home. Some youth may be talkative and pepper family with questions. Others will be less cooperative and more demanding of attention than usual. This can be challenging for families because teens can become difficult as they seek out attention through acting out. However, undesired behavior can serve an important role. It forces engagement, which causes grieving families to regroup.

> Henry is a 12-year-old who just learned that his dad's cancer returned. Henry had been a constant source of support and humor during his father's first and second treatment regimens. When his mom and dad told him that his dad would have to restart medicines and travel to another city for treatment, he responded with irritation: *"OK, fine. So who is going to take me to baseball practice?"* His parents understood that Henry had enough understanding to know that this was very bad news, but at that moment he couldn't take it all in, process yet another loss of his father to cancer, and know that he would have to bear another loss of "normal life." Mostly, he felt deeply scared, and his parents knew that when he was ready, at random times, he would ask the questions that were difficult to speak out loud: *"Is Dad really ever going to get better?"* or *"Is Dad going to die?"* But for now, it made sense that Henry wanted to know how to keep going on with his life and manage this difficult news in small increments.

Older adolescents (about ages 15–17) tend to experience grief in ways more similar to adults. They often have intense emotions, such as sadness and despair, that interfere with normal functioning. Because they are able to think more abstractly, they have a better sense of the permanence of death and also understand the implications that the loss will continue to have on their own life. They mourn specific aspects of their relationship with the deceased, but also mourn the loss of how that relationship would have evolved over time. For instance, teens may say things like, *"Who is going to help me move into my dorm room?"* or *"Who is going to be there when my first child is born?"* Older adolescents also worry about their own mortality in light of the current death. They become intensely focused on things such as the heritability of medical conditions from which their loved ones suffered. In contrast to younger adolescents who tend to focus almost exclusively on themselves, older adolescents have a greater ability to empathize with others suffering around them. They tend to be more willing to spend time with family following a loss. However, they still struggle to find balance between their own needs and caring for other family members. They turn to friends and intimate partners for support, but are still keenly aware of the possibility of rejection from their peer group.

Many teens will also experience sleep disruption. For some, this will manifest as difficulty falling asleep. Teens may lie awake trying to process their loss; others will have nightmares. Nightmares can be related to the actual death or may bring forth other unrelated fears. Sleep difficulties make it hard for teens to get the rest needed to cope with stress.

Adolescents will often test parental boundaries following a loss. They may talk back or refuse to do chores. They may stay out late with friends or experiment with alcohol or drugs. These behaviors serve as an escape from their emotional reality. They also challenge caregivers to set limits. Adolescents are seeking out adults that can reinforce family structures that may have been disrupted by the loss.

Some adolescents will regress. Rather than participating in peer activities, they may wish to spend all of their time with family. For instance, a 16-year-old who used to enjoy going on school trips, playing soccer with a community team, and sleeping overnight at friends' houses may instead now want to stay home. Or a younger adolescent may refuse to go to school. Teens may act younger in a hope that adults around them will focus more on taking care of them. While their behavior can seem childlike, it is a mechanism for coping with emotional intensity; they shut out feelings to attempt to return to a simpler emotional state. They may also be so distraught that they cannot fully participate in activities in which they typically excel.

Sometimes withdrawal from activities may stem from a heightened sense of responsibility to take care of family members, especially if caregivers are so fraught with grief that they are unable to perform their traditional family roles: *"Are they going to be okay? Are they too depressed? Do they need help? Who will take care of my younger siblings if I go out?"*

■ Guilt Is a Normal Part of Grieving

Some adolescents, especially younger teens, grapple with guilt. Younger children may worry they caused a parent's death because they had wished their parent was dead once when they were arguing. Adolescents have a more nuanced sense of guilt. They may think things such as, *"Even though this does not fully make sense, is there a part of me that caused this to happen? If I hadn't been such a pain at home, then maybe she would have gone to the doctor sooner."* Guilt helps explain the loss they have experienced; by giving themselves a role, they find a way to take charge of the situation.

■ Grieving Takes Time

Losing a loved one is life-altering and it takes time to rebuild a network of meaningful relationships. During their initial stages of coping, many adolescents busy themselves with activities, fully immersing themselves in their former lives. This can create confusion for adults, who assume they must not be grieving because they are able to carry on. Adults may say, *"Look how great she is doing. She is still getting straight 'As' and playing varsity soccer."* But, grieving can be extremely unpredictable. Emotions come forth at unexpected moments for months or even years. For instance, a teen may be excited about prom for weeks and beam with joy as she steps out in a new dress. However, when the band plays a song that her ill mother would not allow her to listen to, she may burst into tears and race home. Teens can become incapacitated by grief without notice. Eventually, the unpredictable nature of their grief lessens as adolescents come to terms with the loss.

Emily is a 15-year-old who comes to see you because she can't stop crying. She learned that she has to go on a gluten-free diet and says, *"This is too, too much, I can't do it."* You know Emily to be a practical young person who rarely gets shaken by challenges. So you ask what else is going on. Her mother and best friend, who have both come to the visit, mention Jamie. Emily sits with tears streaming down her face. Jamie, her boyfriend for the last year, broke up with her through a text and told her that he was seeing another girl. Emily couldn't talk. She just teared. When you spend time alone with her, you learn that she can't believe this is happening. She doesn't know what she will do. You ask if she has thoughts of not wanting to be here or wanting to hurt herself or be dead. She clearly says no: *"Who would take care of my younger brothers and my mom?"* You can see that she really doesn't have words to describe how much pain she is in, and you ask her if she remembers being in this much pain before and she responds, *"Only when Daddy died."* and she begins to cry harder. You ask her if she might be having "pain on top of pain" or "piggyback pain." That is, when one loss brings up the memories and deep sadness of an earlier loss. She cries and says all she is dreaming about is her dad. She explains that she was only 10 when he died. Her mom was so sad that Emily started helping around the house and getting the boys off to school. Her mom cried most of that time and struggled to find a job to support the 3 kids. I asked Emily if there was any chance that she could take some time to be sad for the loss of Jamie, but also mourn, more like an adult, the loss of her dad. She looked so relieved. Finally, the "over the top" feelings about breaking up with Jamie (she adds at this point in the conversation that he was really not the best boyfriend) make sense, and Emily starts to share with you (with tears and a little laughter) some funny stories about her dad, whom she hadn't talked about with anyone in a long time.

■ Grief Builds Life Skills

While dealing with loss is one of life's greatest challenges, it also creates opportunity. It is important to remember that grieving adolescents are learning an essential life skill: how to survive loss. As they grieve, they develop a deeper understanding of their emotions. They come to understand their profound capacity for love. And they ultimately find that despite the depth of sadness, they are able to heal and again find joy. These are profound life lessons that carry forth into adulthood. Adolescents must have the room and the support to move through this process so they can become stronger, compassionate adults.

■ Assessment of the Grieving Adolescent

Caring for adolescents who are grieving is an extremely important part of participating in someone's life and helping them move forward. Being able to explore their unique experiences while also helping them understand what is normative is one of the gifts you can give to youth as they heal. Caring adults can support young people by asking questions, listening deeply to their experience, and providing guidance.

- When speaking with grieving youth, it is essential to acknowledge the loss. Acknowledge that grief is an individual experience. Let the adolescent know that you are here to support him or her through the process.
- Take time to explore the adolescent's relationship to the person. Ask about what they enjoyed doing together, a favorite memory, a special personality trait. While some teens may shut down or act angry, others will open up and reveal incredible stories that provide you with a glimpse into their loss. By creating the space for storytelling you allow the adolescent permission to speak openly. By actively listening, you can start to forge a trusting bond that is essential for the healing process.

- It can be very helpful to discuss common symptoms of grief. Let them know that it is normal to feel angry, devastated, guilty, lonely, numb, or indifferent. It is acceptable to not want to deal with it now. Prepare them to feel many different ways over the coming weeks; it is common to have feelings of sadness emerge unexpectedly.
- Understand how the loss has impacted their functioning. Are they going to school? Are they still participating in sports? Have they changed peer groups? Are they able to do things they still enjoy? Are they spending more time alone? Have they been using substances to help cope? Have they made any decisions about relationships or their bodies that they regret? Do they have someone they can talk to about their loss?
- Talk about physical complaints. The mind and body are inherently linked. As adolescents grieve, they often suffer with headaches, abdominal pain, fatigue, chest pain, and insomnia (with or without upsetting dreams) and literally feel that they have a "broken heart." These symptoms can be disabling, especially if they are similar to symptoms experienced by the deceased. Adolescents may worry that they, too, are suffering from a serious affliction (like the lupus that just took their aunt's life). Taking their symptoms seriously and providing reassurance empowers adolescents to understand their body's physical response to grief. Offer advice about the importance of sleep, exercise, a well-balanced diet, and social interaction to help guide them through the healing process.
- Ask about how the loss has changed family functioning. *"Losing someone puts tremendous stress on the whole family. How have things changed in your family since your dad moved out?"* This allows you to assess the degree of dysfunction within the grieving family as well as identify caregivers who may be coping well.
- Ask adolescents if they have suffered previous losses. Listening to discussions about coping with previous loss provides invaluable information about an individual's understanding of grief and the skills he or she developed through the process.
- Identify supportive adults. Ask, *"Who in your life can help you through this?"* Explore whom the teen has reached out to already and brainstorm other potential sources of strength within their network. Ask if it would be helpful for you to speak to these family members, or for you all to meet together, to discuss the healing process.
- Next, it is essential to understand the depth of their loss. Adolescents grappling with acute grief are all struggling to manage their emotions. Care providers must determine which adolescents require immediate professional support due to the severity of their grief experience. Becoming familiar with normal grieving responses as well as signs of more serious disorders is essential (Table 5.1). Are they feeling so sad and confused that they cannot participate in life? Are they wishing they were with the person who is gone? Are they wishing to be dead themselves? These are adolescents who need immediate professional help to ensure they remain safe.

■ Guiding the Youth Toward Help

Many adolescents in the throes of grief will be reluctant to seek help. Care providers should emphasize that seeking help is a sign of personal strength.

> *"Sometimes when you are grieving, you might feel that life will never get better, or even is not worth living. That is the time to get help. Help is a way to go through a path of grieving, to map it out, to accept all of the difficulties, and to move forward in a way that is helpful for you and those around you. It is hard work. It takes incredible strength. Those who do it are brave."* Provide adolescents with support to know that their strength will serve themselves and others. *"You need to do it for yourself, you need to do it for the person who passed away, and you need to do it for the rest of your family."*

Table 5.1

Range of Common Grief Manifestations in Children and Adolescents[a]

Normal or Variant Behavior	Sign of Problem or Disorder[b]
Shock or numbness	Long-term denial and avoidance of feelings
Crying	Repeated crying spells
Sadness	Disabling depression and suicidal ideation
Anger	Persistent anger
Feeling guilty	Believing guilty
Transient unhappiness	Persistent unhappiness
Keeping concerns inside	Social withdrawal
Increased clinging	Separation anxiety
Disobedience	Oppositional or conduct disorder
Lack of interest in school	Decline in school performance
Transient sleep disturbance	Persistent sleep problems
Physical complaints	Physical symptoms of deceased
Decreased appetite	Eating disorder
Temporary regression	Disabling or persistent regression
Being good or bad	Being much too good or bad
Believing deceased is still alive	Persistent belief that deceased is still alive
Adolescent relating better to friends than to family	Promiscuity or delinquent behavior
Behavior lasts days to weeks	Behavior lasts weeks to months

[a]Reprinted with permission from American Academy of Pediatrics Committee on Psychosocial Aspects of Child and Family Health. The pediatrician and childhood bereavement. *Pediatrics.* 2000;105(2):445–447.
[b]Should prompt investigation; mental health referral is recommended.

Adolescents in crisis may have difficulty identifying supportive people. Find out who has helped them through previous stressful times. *"When you are looking for someone to help you get through grief, it is really important you find someone you are comfortable speaking to. You need somebody who has been through it and who you trust, someone who is older and can give you their wisdom."* Help adolescents explore their relationships with parents, grandparents, adult siblings, aunts and uncles, family friends, teachers, school counselors, coaches, and health care professionals. *"Who do you think will be the most helpful for you? When will you have a chance to talk?"* For adolescents you identified as high risk, formulate a plan to ensure prompt follow-up with a mental health professional to ensure their safety.

■ Helping Families Support Grieving Adolescents

Surviving loss puts tremendous stress on families. Parents attempt to support their children while simultaneously grappling with their own grief. It is important for parents to maintain expected family roles to the best of their abilities. Parents should maintain routines and discipline. They should be prepared to de-escalate conflicts that often arise between grieving family members. Teens often feel abandoned and alone following the death of a loved one. Being surrounded by others who are working to maintain a supportive family environment can be extremely healing. It is helpful for parents to identify other adults who can step up to handle family responsibilities if the parent is too overwhelmed by grief.

Honesty is essential to help families move forward. Encourage parents to openly discuss the circumstances surrounding the loss. Parents often want to shield their children from death, hoping to lessen the grief they experience. However, adolescents understand death and feel betrayed when adults are being secretive. Allow teens to ask questions and answer them as openly as possible.

Help parents understand that adolescent grief looks different from adult grief. Anger is often very pronounced and can be directed at surviving family members. Regressive behavior is common. Teens often have erratic emotions in the weeks to months following a death, with emotions emerging at unexpected moments. It is important that parents create a safe space for teens to express their emotions. Younger adolescents, who are often embarrassed by public displays of emotion, may benefit from more structured times to reminisce. Bringing the family together to do an activity that was meaningful to the deceased provides a wonderful opportunity to share memories.

Parents need to be mindful that just because their teen has resumed activity as usual and seems to be coping well, they are still working through profound suffering. Older adolescents often feel that they must "keep it together" for the sake of the family; they worry that, if they take time to grieve, their family will fall apart. Parents need to be alert to this tendency and make sure that teens know it is all right for them to work through their own grief. This may mean that teens miss several days of school, do not keep up their grades, or decline trying out for the soccer team. Grieving teens are participating in an incredible project. That project is learning about loss and about surviving loss. When we expect adolescents to bypass normal emotions so they can keep getting As in school, we will have foregone immeasurably important life lessons. We will have set up unrealistic expectations and will not have helped them develop into strong, resilient adults.

Participating in bereavement rituals can be very healing. Offer adolescents the opportunity to participate in memorial services. Find out what portions of the services they wish to attend, but do not force them to join if they do not want to. Many teens will want to pay tribute to their loved one by speaking, reading a poem, or creating a photo montage. Other teens will find more solace through personal journal writing. Reflecting on treasured memories is an important part of the healing process. Parents should be sure to honor their child's individual approach to grieving while providing opportunities to mourn with others in their community.

Help parents identify supportive peers. By late adolescence, peers are a strong source of emotional support. Parents can help identify trusted friends to be present through the grief process. This allows grieving adolescents to continue on their developmental trajectories. Having emotional outlets outside of the family can also help reduce conflict within the family.

Inform family members of the warning signs of severe grief. Parents know their children best, so they are well poised to seek help for their struggling teen. Discuss that it is very common for adolescents to struggle following a loss. Assess parental willingness to seek help from a health professional and provide resources so that parents feel empowered to help their teen. Discuss referral for professional counseling for teens exhibiting severe symptoms. Research suggests that participation in structured psycho-educational support groups can improve outcomes for both adolescents and parents.

Encourage parents to care for themselves. Parents may be so focused on protecting others that they do not meet their own basic needs, let alone process their own loss. Reassure parents that it is not selfish to care for themselves; indeed it is a strategic act of good parenting. Explain that children respond to adversity best when their parents remain stable and serve as models for healthy coping.

■ A Path Forward

There are many different ways to work through grief. Some of it is time. Some of it is talking with family, trusted adults, and health care professionals. Some of it is getting back to usual activities and busying oneself. Sometimes it is a feeling that you are fulfilling a mission of the person who passed away by doing something in their honor.

Care providers play a fundamental role in helping youth move forward. By creating a safe environment to explore grief and listening to adolescents' stories, they can begin the healing process. Youth often describe a feeling of emptiness following a loss. They seek various strategies to fill this void. Some of these strategies, such as alcohol and drug use and sexual promiscuity, put vulnerable teens in high-risk situations that can jeopardize their futures. Steering teens toward positive strategies, in contrast, strengthens their repertoire of coping mechanisms.

Justin is a 17-year-old who came into the office for a routine physical. He wore a baseball cap that cast a long shadow over his forehead as he sat slumped in an examination room chair. His eyes fixed on the floor as he answered questions about his medical history with short sentences. We eventually moved on to discuss his social history. I asked, *"Whom do you live with?"* The question, which for most adolescents serves as a harmless introduction to discuss more sensitive topics, hung heavy in the air. *"It's complicated,"* he shrugged. I asked, *"What does complicated look like?"* He discussed how he had been bouncing around between foster families for the past 2 years. *"I move around a lot because I keep getting in fights."* When I asked him what made him angry enough to fight, he said, *"People are always messing with me, talking s**t about me."* He revealed that he was suspended from school for fighting and on the verge of being kicked out of his district. I asked him who he used to live with before entering foster care. He described how his father left when Justin was very young and his mother has been in and out of rehab for alcohol and heroin use. *"Was there anyone in your family you used to be close to?"* I inquired. *"My grandmother was always there for me. She took me in and raised me while my mom was away. She took good care of me, made sure I had a good home-cooked dinner, was always nagging me to do my homework, made sure I pressed my shirt for church on Sunday morning...."* His voice trailed off and then he said, *"But she is dead now. Died of cancer a few years ago. And my mom, she didn't even come to the funeral. Only thing she gives a d**n about is getting high. And so I had nowhere to go."* After a pause I said, *"I can tell you loved your grandmother deeply. What do you think it was about her that made her so special?"* As he told stories of his grandmother teaching Sunday school, bringing neighborhood kids into her home who were in search of a warm meal, picking up trash that littered the sidewalk, and gathering old winter coats to donate to a local shelter, Justin's eyes lit up. For the first time during our visit, he cracked a small smile. *"And it's just not right that she is gone while all these other losers are still hanging around in the neighborhood,"* he said. *"Your grandmother sounds like she was an amazing person, and I can tell that her death was tremendously hard. What do you think she would say if she were here now?"* He sat silently for a while, and then said softly, *"She'd tell me I gotta keep going and I can't give up."* I reflected to him that he had already shown a tremendous amount of strength to move forward. I asked him what he wanted to do with his life and he said, *"I want to be a counselor to help kids when they hit rough spots."* I looked him right in the eye and said, *"Your grandmother would be so proud."* He allowed himself to cry.

From there, we talked about how fighting could get in the way of his desire to honor his grandmother's memory. We came up with strategies he could use to get out of fights. And we figured out that he could volunteer at a local library helping neighborhood kids with their homework. By listening to the story of his loss and helping him figure out how to pay tribute to his grandmother through his actions, Justin was able to move forward.

Assisting adolescents in honoring the legacy of lost loved ones can be healing. It allows them to take charge. It allows them to channel their feelings in a positive direction. Creative expression is another powerful tool to promote healing 5.1 following a loss. Journal writing, poetry writing, and drawing give adolescents a safe space to express their emotions. They may choose to share portions of their work with family, friends, or caring professionals, or they may choose to keep their expressions private. Youth are often surprised by the power of their own words. They are able to explore the depths of their sadness and relive bittersweet memories. Creative outlets allow them to begin to move forward to become compassionate and resilient adults.

●● Group Learning and Discussion ●●

1. Prior to this session, assign one member of the group to find local resources for grieving youth.
2. Discuss the wide range of ways youth in grief have presented in your practice setting.
3. Break into pairs and choose a case in which a youth "acted out" to deal with her grief, sought revenge, or even her own death as a means to handle her emotions. If you do not have a case, use one of the 2 below. Guide these youth toward channeling their grief by honoring the legacy of those they have lost.
   a. Cicely is a 14-year-old who has recently lost her grandmother. She has argued incessantly with her mother recently. She implores, *"I am nothing like her!"* She palpably misses her grandmother, whom she visited weekly at the elder community. Her grandmother always showed her off to all of her friends, and she used to even play cards with them. She tearfully says that she wishes she could be with her grandmother.
   b. Shane comes into the community center and things just seem different. He is irritable and seems to intentionally foul the other men on the court. The youth worker takes him aside and comments that something seems to be on his mind. He fumes, *"D**n straight I'm angry. My cousin was shot and he has a little girl. Just a baby. He wanted to be a cop. Showed off her picture all the time, had big dreams for her. She's never gonna know him. It's alright though, I'll find out who did it."*

■ Related Video Content ▶

5.0 Supporting Youth Through the Grieving Process. Kinsman.

5.1 Dealing With Grief by Living Life More Purposefully. Ginsburg.

■ Related Resources

American Academy of Child and Adolescent Psychiatry
Facts for Families: Children and Grief. http://www.aacap.org/cs/root/facts_for_families/children_and_grief
> This information sheet reviews common grief symptoms and behavioral manifestations. It highlights concerning symptoms for which parents should seek help from mental health professionals.

American Academy of Pediatrics
Addressing Mental Health Concerns in Primary Care: A Clinician's Toolkit
http://tinyurl.aap.org/pub112382
> This toolkit provides up-to-date management advice, care plans, documentation and coding advice, parent handouts, and community resources to help address a variety of mental health concerns including grief, depression, anxiety, attention issues, substance use, learning differences, and other mental health concerns.

American Academy of Pediatrics Committee on Psychosocial Aspects of Child and Family Health. The pediatrician and childhood bereavement. *Pediatrics*. 2000;105(2):445–447
> This article reviews children and adolescents' response to grief and provides guidance for pediatricians to use when caring for patients and families following a loss.

HealthyChildren.org
www.healthychildren.org/EmotionalWellness
> This site focuses on helping parents promote emotional wellness across all ages.

Christ GH, Siegel K, Christ AE. Adolescent grief. "It never really hit me…until it finally happened." *JAMA*. 2002;288(10):1269–1278
> This article uses a teen's narrative to explore developmental models of grief, with a specific focus on coping with loss in relation to a terminally ill parent. It provides age-specific helpful strategies for engaging youth throughout the illness, death, and mourning periods.

Christ GH. Impact of development on children's mourning. *Cancer Pract*. 2000;8(2):72–81
> The author uses a qualitative approach to analyze interviews with grieving children and then highlights features of the grief response across the age spectrum. The article specifically discusses what grief looks like, what parental attributes are mourned, key developmental characteristics, and parental tasks to facilitate coping in 5 different age groups.

Dehlin L, Martensson L. Adolescents' experiences of a parent's serious illness and death. *Palliat Support Care*. 2009;7:13–25
> This qualitative study uses interviews with grieving teens to describe the threat of parental death, how adolescents manage this threat, and how they cope with loneliness following death. It includes multiple interview excerpts that allow teens to describe the grieving process in their own words.

Kubler-Ross E, Kessler D. *On Grief and Grieving: Finding the Meaning of Grief Through the Five Stages of Loss*. New York, NY: Scribner; 2007
> This book builds on the author's classic *On Death and Dying*, which changed the way we talk about death. It added understanding on the grieving process.

Kirwin KM, Hamrin V. Decreasing the risk of complicated bereavement and future psychiatric disorders in children. *J Child Adolesc Psychiatr Nurs*. 2005;18(2):62–78
> This article synthesizes various theoretical models of grieving and explores psychological factors that affect the grieving process. It outlines the importance of support from families and care providers to improve long-term mental health outcomes for grieving youth.

Lancaster J. Developmental stages, grief, and a child's response to death. *Pediatr Ann*. 2011;40(5):277–281
> This article examines the stages of grief through a developmental lens. It also discusses myths surrounding childhood grief and risk/protective factors that impact bereavement.

Moreno M, Furtner F, Rivara F. Advice for patients: when a loved one dies. *Arch Pediatr Adolesc Med*. 2012;166(3):296
> This patient handout explains children's and adolescents' response to grief and provides concrete tips parents can use to help their families after a loss.

Riely M. Facilitating children's grief. *J Sch Nurs*. 2003;19(4):212–218

> This article focuses on the role of school health professionals in guiding children through the grieving process. It provides suggestions for school-based therapeutic interventions and outlines guidelines and resources for implementing grief support programs for children and families.

Substance Abuse and Mental Health Services Administration
www.samhsa.gov/MentalHealth/Anxiety_Grief.pdf

> This informational handout for patients provides basic information about grief as well as online resources.

Strategies to Help Youth Cope With Challenges

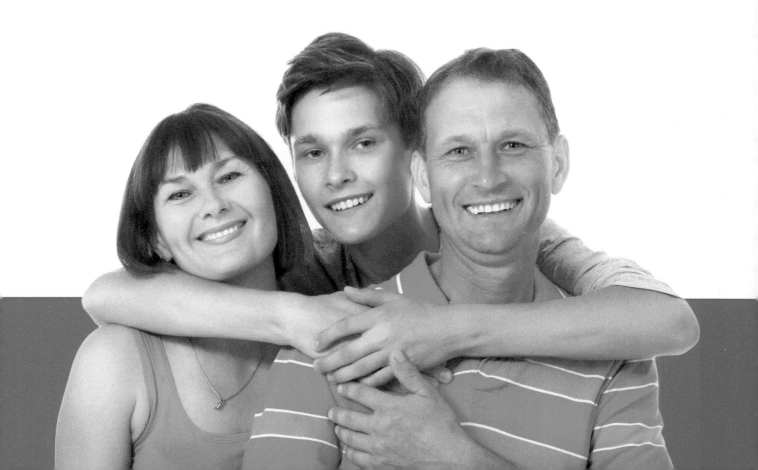

CHAPTER 6

Health Realization—Accessing a Higher State of Mind No Matter What

Nimi Singh, MD, MPH, MA

 Related Video Content

6.0 Achieving a State of Optimal Health: Stress and the Health Realization Model

■ Why This Matters

Teaching adolescents to increase their ability to cope with stress optimizes physical and psychological well-being, strengthens decision-making, and leads to positive social interactions and improved school performance.

> **By becoming aware of the quality of our thinking and disengaging from negative thoughts, we can learn to shut off our stress response and think more clearly.**

■ Stress Response and Its Effect on the Mind

The stress response allows us to perceive a potential environmental threat to our survival. It triggers a physiological response that allows us to get ourselves to safety quickly, by either fighting a potential predator, fleeing, or freezing and blending unnoticed into the environment. Each of these actions requires providing those parts of the body critical for fighting, fleeing, or even freezing with a sudden burst of energy. This is achieved by the shunting of blood to vital organs so oxygen and nutrients are delivered to the heart, lungs, muscles, and our brain stem, the part of the brain that controls heart rate, breathing rate, and temperature. As blood shunts to these organs and tissues, it shunts away from those organs *not* critical for survival, namely the digestive system, the reproductive system, the immune system, and the prefrontal cortex, that part of the brain that provides "executive functioning," including abstract thinking and creative problem-solving, that allows us to see the "big picture." In other words, our highest cognitive functioning is impaired as those bodily systems not critical for survival-in-the-moment become relatively compromised. In parallel, our bodies don't function well when the stress response is chronically firing in response to real or perceived challenges.

We are most prepared to deal with life's challenges when our bodies and minds are functioning in a healthy, integrated manner.

Unfortunately, the stress response gets triggered just as easily in the face of a mis-perceived threat to our survival as it does to a true threat. Even remembering negative thoughts about the past, as well as having worries about the future can trigger this survival mechanism. These thoughts are not true threats to our survival, but our body doesn't know this!

Stress causes our minds to perceive the world through a lens of increased arousal, alertness, and vigilance, where every stimulus in the environment is misperceived as a potential threat to our survival. While this can be life-saving in truly dangerous circumstances, it hinders our ability to think clearly in other situations. As blood flow shunts away from the higher-functioning areas of our brains to our brain stems (also called the "reptilian" brain), we can experience our minds going "blank" when we try to retrieve stored information. In this state, we also become unable to take in and easily process new information. This can lead to distorted or "negative thinking." Chronic repetitive, negative thoughts about the future can increase anxiety. Negative thoughts about the past (eg, anger, sadness, shame, regret, guilt) can contribute to depression. Harmful coping mechanisms or addictive behaviors (eg, substance use or cutting) can be understood as attempts to minimize stress and "quiet the mind" of negative thoughts (see Chapter 8).

What's extraordinary about our consciousness is the fact that the mind has an innate ability to *self-right;* that is, disengage from negative thoughts and return to present-moment thinking. When this occurs, it allows the blood flow to shunt back to the prefrontal cortex, the seat of higher cognitive functioning. Most of the time this happens automatically, but sometimes we get stuck in "stress mode." In order to facilitate the mind's ability to self-right, we need to understand what helps to shut off the stress response.

■ Shutting Off the Stress Response

Critical first steps in optimizing our ability to let go of negative thoughts, and, therefore, shut off the stress response, include good sleep hygiene, optimal nutrition, and adequate physical activity (see Chapter 7). Learning self-regulatory techniques, such as progressive muscle relaxation, deep breathing, and mental imagery (also known as self-hypnosis), is also helpful, as are other forms of biobehavioral training, such as using biofeedback machines and programs. Inviting adolescents struggling with stress to reconnect with recreational activities that they enjoy also helps reduce baseline stress levels over time.

Body movement therapies, such as yoga, have been shown in clinical studies to reduce stress and improve mental and physical functioning. Finally, psychotherapies that fall under the category of "cognitive behavioral therapies" teach people struggling with anxiety and depression that stress-based thinking is faulty thinking, and that they can learn to notice their own negative thoughts and choose to ignore or override them. Health realization, one form of this type of therapy, focuses on the mind's innate capacity to self-right simply by noticing the quality of one's thinking.

■ Health Realization

Health realization explores healthy psychological functioning: what it looks like, what gets in its way, and what we can do about it. We can train ourselves to get into the habit of noticing our own negative thoughts, disengaging from them, and thus shifting to a higher state of functioning. It reminds us that

• We are the creators of our own thoughts.
• The quality of our thinking (positive, negative, or neutral) creates our perception of reality in the moment.
• Negative thoughts trigger our stress response, which distorts our perceptions and yields unreliable and inaccurate information.

By becoming aware of the quality of our thinking and disengaging from negative thoughts, we can learn to shut off our stress response and think more clearly.

■ Understanding Our Thoughts Better

Estimates of how many individual thoughts the average person has in a given day range from 40,000 to 60,000. Most are old thoughts we've had over and over again. Furthermore, these repetitive thoughts tend to be either worries about the future or anger/sadness/regret/shame/guilt about the past. If we allow ourselves to repeat these thoughts, we trigger our stress physiology and impair our physical and psychological functioning.

Physical stresses, such as being tired, hungry, or ill, increase our awareness of these old thoughts. One way to mitigate this is to be aware of what is needed to restore optimal functioning (eg, restful sleep, healthy nutrition, exercise, and focusing on self-care).

Two Modes of Thought

We can consider 2 modes of thought. The first is "left-brain" or "conditioned mode," which is associated with accessing stored information, computation, and comparison, and can be likened to being in "computer" mode. Our state of mind in this mode tends to be busy and mechanical. This is useful when we're exploring situations that have only one right answer. The second mode is "right-brain" or "exploratory" thinking, which is associated with creativity, insight, inspiration, and accessing one's own wisdom and common sense, and can be likened to being in "receiver mode." In this "exploratory mode," our state of mind tends to be more calm and peaceful, and this is useful in situations when there is no one "right" answer. We get into trouble when we're in "conditioned mode" when we should be in "exploratory mode." "Exploratory mode" helps us interact positively with others, understand new or different points of view, or expand our thinking beyond what we already know. When we find ourselves interacting ineffectively with others, we can learn to notice if we're accidentally seeing the person through "old thoughts" about who we think they are. We are likely to find these old thoughts are keeping us from interacting in a fresh, unbiased, and exploratory manner. This realization can ultimately create a new dynamic of interaction.

■ Moods

Moods, like thoughts, come and go. It's helpful to think of moods as being "high" or "low," rather than "good" or "bad." This takes the judgment out of our observations. Our moods can affect the quality of our thinking (eg, low moods cause stress and distorted thoughts) and can themselves be created by the thoughts we're entertaining (eg, negative thoughts create a low mood). Just like thoughts, moods can be affected by one's physical state. Fatigue, illness, or a stressful event can bring on a "low" mood. Some people's moods can be affected by what they eat, what chemicals they're exposed to in the environment, even the weather.

We can't always change the mood we're in, but we can learn to notice our mood and try and support ourselves to minimize the effects of the mood on our functioning. Being aware of moods can help one understand others. Others may behave poorly at times due to a low mood or negative thinking, which distorts how they're seeing and interacting with the world. If their mood were higher, they'd see the world more clearly and make better choices.

This allows us, as professionals, to see the blamelessness and innocence of others. When communicating with someone in a stressful situation, try to notice your own mood, quiet your own thinking, and just observe. Listen carefully and with understanding.

Remember that you can project feelings of warmth and safety, which will help the other person feel more secure, shut off their stress response, and, therefore, raise the quality of their thinking.

Guidelines Around Moods

Recognize Moods

- Assess your mood level and that of others.
- Recognize how thoughts can create moods (and let negative thoughts go!).
- Remember: *You* create/sustain moods (inside-out process).
- Be easy on yourself and others.
- "See the innocence!"

Managing a Low Mood

- Develop a way to recognize this in yourself.
- Suspend major decisions until you are coming from a place of calm and security.
- Don't always trust your own thinking.
- Be careful about taking yourself/others too seriously.
- Be cautious of verbal/behavioral interactions.
- Don't commiserate—moods can be infectious!
- Let others know what you need.
- Slow down your thinking (drop, distract, dismiss, and ignore)—**drop** negative thoughts, **distract** yourself away from those thoughts, **dismiss** them as you notice them arise in your mind, and train yourself to **ignore** them when they reappear.
- Pamper yourself.
- Give yourself a time-out.

Separate Realities

Thoughts, along with our past experience, shape our sense of reality. Our view of reality changes moment to moment depending on our emotional state. The "lower" our mood, the more attached we are to our view of reality. The "higher" our mood, the more comfort and tolerance we experience with respect to different realities and points of view. People unknowingly create their reality based on the quality of their moment-to-moment thinking. Further, most people are often unaware how their mood is affecting their thinking. In other words, our thoughts at any given moment *are* what creates our experience and view of reality.

■ When More Is Needed

When supporting someone who is struggling with stress and low moods, there may be signs that they need to be referred to a professional, either for formal cognitive behavioral therapy, medication, or both. These signs include excessive irritability, loss of pleasure in activities, marked weight loss or weight gain, marked change in sleeping habits, difficulty concentrating, low energy, feelings of low self-worth, excessive guilt, or hopelessness. In this situation, assisting the young person in getting a formal mental health evaluation is critical.

•• Group Learning and Discussion ••

In order to most effectively convey the benefits of the health realization model to teens, it may be helpful for you to first experience how it can control your reactions to your own thoughts.

1. Listening exercise

   In order to become more aware of how our minds stay active with intrusive thoughts, even when our role is to simply listen, engage in the following exercise:

   a. Sit in pairs. Each person will spend 3 minutes telling a childhood story to the other person. It can be a happy, sad, or neutral story. The role of the listener is to simply listen. Even if the other person says something that elicits an emotional response in the listener, the listener can notice it but should not act on it. There should be no comments made, conversation, or even gestures made to the other in response to the content, other than simply listening deeply.

   b. After the 3 minutes are done, the storyteller and listener switch roles.

   c. At the end of the exercise, the facilitator asks people to share what it was like to be the storyteller. Then the facilitator asks what it was like to be the listener. The facilitator should acknowledge and validate all responses, since there is a wide range of human reactions to being listened to deeply and to listening deeply.

   d. After the respondents are finished sharing their experiences, the facilitator can gently point out the extent to which we all get caught up in our own thoughts and how that takes us out of being fully present to the other person when we interact with them. The facilitator may also point out how powerful (and sometimes even healing) it is to have someone simply listen to our stories.

2. Separate realities

   a. Have a bath towel available and ask the group if someone is willing to come up and show the group the "proper way" to fold a bath towel. Next ask someone else to show their way if it's different. After 3 or 4 people have shown how they fold bath towels, ask each of them to explain why their way "makes the most sense." The facilitator can then review with the group how we, as human beings, all have our own reasons for doing things the way we do, and they seem "right" to us, even if they seem "wrong" to others. The facilitator may then point out that no one is "right" or "wrong," we simply all have our own "separate realities" based on our life experiences.

■ Suggested Reading

Claypatch C. Articulating health realization in a nutshell (monograph). Minneapolis, MN: Glenwood-Lyndale Health Realization Training Center; 2005

Folkman S. Positive psychological states and coping with severe stress. *Soc Sci Med.* 2006;45:1207

Halcon L, Robertson CL, Monsen KA, Claypatch CC. A theoretical framework for using health realization to reduce stress and improve coping in refugee communities. *J Holis Nurs.* 2007;25:186–194

Pransky J. *Parenting from the Heart: A Common Sense Approach to Parenting.* Moretown, VT: NEHRI Publications; 2001

■ Related Video Content

6.0 Achieving a State of Optimal Health: Stress and the Health Realization Model. Singh.

CHAPTER 7

The Role of Lifestyle in Mental Health Promotion

Nimi Singh, MD, MPH, MA

 Related Video Content

7.0 The Role of Lifestyle and Healthy Thinking in Mental Health Promotion

■ Why It Matters

Current estimates are that 1 in 5 adolescents will experience a mood disorder at some point before reaching adulthood. There is a substantial body of scientific evidence that, for many individuals, lifestyle and environment (including stress, nutrition, physical activity, and sleep) significantly affect mental functioning[1]. Further, there is growing evidence that addressing these basic issues can play a critical role in restoring mental and emotional well-being. Optimizing lifestyle may be critical to managing stress, anxiety, and depression, as well as other lifestyle-related diseases such as hypertension, dyslipidemias, insulin resistance, metabolic syndrome, and coronary artery disease.

> **A key to improving mental health is remembering "grandmother's wisdom": "Eat your veggies, get enough exercise, go out and play, get enough rest...and take time to relax."**

For all of these reasons, it is critical for us to support youth in restoring their optimal health by addressing these fundamental issues both preventively and as part of our treatment plan for mood disorders and stress in adolescents.

■ Alternative Definitions of Mental Functioning

In light of how stress is known to affect cognition and mood, what if we were to consider anxiety and depression as the temporary loss of the ability to self-right psychologically? The "stress" response keeps getting triggered, producing distorted thinking, uneven moods, and poor behavior (see Chapter 6). Mental health might then be seen as the ability to return to normal functioning after experiencing psychological stress.

■ Treating Psychological Distress

Treating psychological distress, whether anxiety or depression, then can be thought of as optimizing the body's own ability to shut off the stress response and return to optimal functioning. Critical first steps include good sleep hygiene, optimal nutrition, and adequate physical activity. Specific stress-management techniques are also extremely helpful and include self-regulatory techniques, such as progressive muscle relaxation, deep breathing, and mental imagery. Body movement therapies, such as yoga, Tai chi, Qigong, and engaging in enjoyable recreational activities, also all contribute in lowering baseline stress levels and improved coping with stress. Finally, actually learning cognitive behavioral strategies allows one to learn to disengage from and discount negative thoughts. This can be achieved through traditional cognitive behavioral approaches, such as dialectical behavioral therapy, as well as more strength-based strategies, such as health realization and mindfulness-based stress reduction (see chapters 6 and 9).

Screening: The Basics (What to Ask Youth)

Sleep

- *"What's your typical routine before you get into bed?"*
- *"What time do you get in bed?"*
- *"How long does it take for you to fall asleep?"*
- *"Do you stay awake thinking about things? What things?"*
- *"Do you wake up sooner than you want? If yes, is it hard to fall asleep again?"*

Nutrition

Whole foods versus processed foods? Phytonutrient intake (dark leafy greens, colorful fruits and vegetables)?

Multivitamin, supplements?

Exercise

How often? How much? If not, was there a time when you did?

Body movement therapies (Yoga, Tai chi, Qigong, etc)?

Recreation and Relaxation

Recreational activities (creative vs passive is better, such as art, music, journaling, hobbies, etc...)?

What do you do to relax (familiarity with breathing strategies, meditation, etc)?

Optimizing Homeostasis

Sleep

A 2003 National Survey of Children's Health revealed that 15 million US children and teens get inadequate sleep. This alone has been found to be a risk factor for anxiety and depression. Anxiety and depression, in turn, lead to poor sleep quality and quantity. Optimal hours of regenerative sleep, when cortisol ought to be at its lowest level and growth hormone at its highest, is between 10:00 pm and 2:00 am. Many adolescents miss some or part of this optimal period of sleep. The National Sleep Foundation defines sleep hours for adolescents as inadequate if they receive less than 8 hours per night, borderline if 8 hours per night, and optimal if more than 9 hours per night. Eaton et al[2] looked at the 2007 Youth Risk Behavior Survey and found that almost 70% of adolescents reported getting inadequate sleep, and only 8% reported getting optimal sleep.

What gets in the way of obtaining optimal sleep? School schedules, intellectually stimulating activities (TV, Internet, reading), and caffeine-containing foods and beverages. What helps? Limiting daytime naps, exercising during the day, and optimizing the sleep environment (the room should be quiet, dark, with minimal to no distractions). Having a regular sleep routine, where the last meal or snack is ideally no less than 2 hours before sleeping. ▶ **8.3.4**

Nutrition

There is a growing recognition that, in the United States, much of the population is malnourished. We don't suffer from a macronutrient deficiency (we get enough calories from carbohydrates, proteins, and fats), but rather from a micronutrient deficiency. Micronutrients include vitamins, minerals, and the "phytonutrients" in colorful fruits and vegetables, all of which serve as critical cofactors for the enzymatic processes that allow us to convert carbohydrates, fats, and proteins into energy.

Without an adequate daily supply of these micronutrients, we run the risk of our cells functioning suboptimally, or even malfunctioning. Unfortunately, most Americans have diets high in processed foods, which are depleted in these critical micronutrients. Even foods artificially fortified with vitamins and minerals don't allow the body to absorb those nutrients nearly as efficiently as do whole foods as they occur in nature.

The beneficial, protective anti-inflammatory effects of omega-3 fatty acids are being documented for a wide variety of chronic inflammatory conditions, and are also being recognized as improving response to psychotropic medications, suggesting that, in some cases, anxiety and depression may be, in part, pro-inflammatory states. This could explain, in part, the presumed rise in mood disorders (part of the rise is likely improved help-seeking and reporting), given that other chronic inflammatory conditions are also on the rise (allergies, asthma, eczema, to name a few).

Vitamins found in dark leafy greens, such as thiamine, niacin, pyridoxine, folate, cobalamin, and co-enzyme Q10, are all understood to be critical to nervous system health. All youth with mood disorders (and any chronic inflammatory disorder, for that matter) should be screened for vitamin D deficiency and supplemented as needed. Important minerals that serve in important enzymatic processes include calcium, chromium, iodine, iron, magnesium, selenium, and zinc. For this reason, someone struggling with anxiety or depression may benefit from being started on a good multivitamin as a helpful first step toward improving nutrition, since it is difficult to change one's diet overnight. Over time, however, it's best to slowly increase one's consumption of whole fruits and vegetables as the best way to optimize cell functioning.

Finally, timing of food is also very important. A 2005 study by Mahoney and colleagues[3] demonstrated a relationship between breakfast composition and cognitive functioning in elementary school children. Breakfast should optimally include protein plus complex carbohydrate plus essential fatty acids (omega-3 fatty acids). These were found to help in maintaining focus, producing higher-quality work, and improving mood. Skipping meals such as breakfast creates the risk of developing low blood sugar, with the result of increased hunger, overeating, a spike in insulin, and subsequent low blood sugar, starting the cycle over again. Smaller, more frequent meals, alternatively, are associated with a more steady supply of glucose to brain. ▶ **8.3.3**

Physical Activity

A growing number of studies have linked exercise with beneficial effects on mental health. Purported mechanisms of action include increased release of dopamine, the neurotransmitter associated with pleasure and happy moods, increased blood flow, increasing oxygen and nutrients to the brain, reduced inflammation, altering brain wave activity, and increasing restful sleep, to name a few. Research has found positive effects for the following specific types of exercises: aerobic activity (including brisk walking), strength training, and yoga.

As Dr Kathi Kemper suggests in her 2010 book, *Mental Health Naturally*,[1] the best exercise is one the individual enjoys and will maintain over time. Ideally, it should occur 3 to 5 times a week, 20 to 30 minutes at a minimum. There is evidence to suggest that we get most benefit from exercise in the first 30 minutes, so that is a perfectly reasonable goal for most people.

8.3.1

Recreational Activities

Finally, we often discount the value of encouraging adolescents to engage in hobbies, have some quiet unstructured time, spend time in nature, and engage in some form of creative activity or play. Passive entertainment, such as watching TV, does not engage the brain in the same beneficial way as the activities mentioned above.

•• Group Learning and Discussion ••

Mental, emotional, and behavioral health are often considered the "new morbidity," as they drive so many problems. Discuss as a group whether you tend to be more reactive to these problems or whether you have also incorporated prevention into your approach. If not, consider how to most effectively promote wellness in your setting. View the materials associated with this chapter to see some strategies on how to present the importance of sleep, exercise, nutrition, and relaxation. Then consider how to convey these points in a way that would be most helpful to the teens you serve.

■ References

1. Kemper KJ. *Mental Health Naturally: The Family Guide to Holistic Care for a Healthy Mind and Body.* Elk Grove Village, IL: American Academy of Pediatrics; 2010
2. Eaton DK, McKnight-Eily LR, Lowry R, Perry GS, Presley-Cantrell L, Croft JB. Prevalence of insufficient, borderline and optimal hours of sleep among high school students—United States. *J Adolesc Health.* 2010;46(4):399–401
3. Mahoney CR, Taylor HA, Kanarek RB, Samuel P. Effect of breakfast composition on cognitive processes in elementary school children. *Physiol Behav.* 2005;85(5):635–645

■ Suggested Reading

Beasley PJ, Beardslee WR. Depression in adolescent patients. *Adolesc Med.* 1998;9(2):351–362

Birmaher B, Ryan ND, Williamson DE, Brent DA, Kaufman J. Childhood and adolescent depression: a review of the past ten years. *J. Am Acad Child Adolesc Psychiatry.* 1996;35(12):1575–1583

Brown S. *Play: How it Shapes the Brain, Opens the Imagination and Invigorates the Soul.* New York, NY: Penguin; 2010

Hamrin V, Magorno M. Assessment of adolescents for depression in the pediatric primary care setting: diagnostic criteria and clinical manifestations of depression in adolescents. *Pediatr Nurs.* 2010;36(2):103–111

Hyman M. *The UltraMind Solution.* New York, NY: Scribner; 2010

Murphy JM, Pagano ME, Nachmani J, et al. The relationship of school breakfast to psychosocial and academic functioning: cross-sectional and longitudinal observations in an inner-city school sample. *Arch Pediatr Adolesc Med.* 1998;152(9):899–907

Ratey JJ, Hagerman E. *Spark: The Revolutionary New Science of Exercise and the Brain.* New York, NY: Little, Brown and Company; 2008

■ Related Video Content ▶

7.0 The Role of Lifestyle and Healthy Thinking in Mental Health Promotion. Singh.

8.3.1 Stress Management and Coping/Section 2/Taking Care of My Body/Point 4: The Power of Exercise. Ginsburg.

8.3.2 Stress Management and Coping/Section 2/Taking Care of My Body/Point 5: Active Relaxation. Ginsburg.

8.3.3 Stress Management and Coping/Section 2/Taking Care of My Body/Point 6: Eat Well. Ginsburg.

8.3.4 Stress Management and Coping/Section 2/Taking Care of My Body/Point 7: Sleep Well. Ginsburg.

CHAPTER 8

Stress Management and Coping

Kenneth R. Ginsburg, MD, MS Ed, FAAP, FSAHM

 Related Video Content

8.0 Stress Management and Coping

■ Why This Matters

The ability to cope with life's stressors in a positive way is key to overcoming adversity.[1] Figure 8.1 illustrates how stress can lead to a variety of outcomes. A life stressor creates discomfort that is reduced by employing a coping strategy. If equipped with positive adaptive strategies, the individual will gain some degree of relief, but maladaptive strategies also offer relief. In fact, many negative coping strategies are quick and easy fixes that offer near-instant relief.[2]

> **Rather than condemning negative behavior, which may only increase stress, we invite youth to join with us in a healing process to build positive coping strategies.**

These quick fixes might be the social morbidities we worry about the most—drinking, drug use, sensation seeking, self-mutilation, sex out of the context of a healthy relationship, truancy, gang affiliation, violence, and running away, among others. All of these strategies offer fleeting relief but lead to troubling patterns. First, stress leads to an unhealthy action that, in turn, may lead to increased tension within the individual, conflict with parents, educational underperformance, or social failures. These added pressures lead to more stress that leads to ever more reliance on the unhealthy fix.

■ Assessing the Stressor

A first step is to accurately assess the stressor. Stress is an adaptive tool that transforms our minds and bodies to react to potentially life-threatening emergencies. A small amount of stress increases our vigilance and prepares us to react. A large amount of stress prepares our body to fight or escape. The problem is that our stress-response system was not designed for the modern world. When a person reacts to a stressor with the same full-blown response he would to a true life or death emergency, it can be maladaptive. When a stressor is experienced out of proportion to its real potential effect, it is known as "catastrophic thinking." If a person is stuck in a pattern of catastrophic thinking, it can lead to ongoing anxiety and hyperreactivity. The first step of accurately assessing the stressor is determining if it is a "real tiger" or a "paper tiger." A worry is not a "real tiger." The next step to avert catastrophic thought is to remember that bad things are often temporary. Once a person considers how he will feel in a week or 2, he can remind himself that he can get through this. Equally as important is to grasp that good things might just be well deserved and can be permanent. Otherwise, people can experience stress even during good

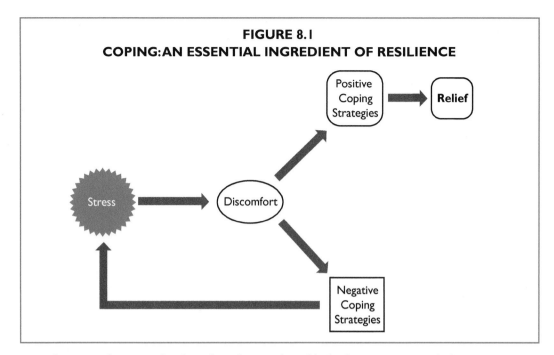

FIGURE 8.1
COPING: AN ESSENTIAL INGREDIENT OF RESILIENCE

times because they wait for the other shoe to drop.[3,4] The best strategy to help coping in those cases where simple reflections will not suffice may be to work on adjusting thinking patterns through cognitive behavioral therapy.[5-7] Healthy thinking patterns are important for reframing negative thoughts that interfere with forward progress.

The coping plan to be presented here is designed to build a repertoire of positive coping strategies so that, in times of inevitable stress, a person will naturally turn to these healthy strategies rather than to the quick, but dangerous, fixes that are termed "negative coping strategies" in this model.

■ Coping: An Essential Component of the Behavioral Change Process

One of the key concepts within Prochaska's[8] transtheoretical model of behavioral change is decisional balance. This involves an individual weighing the costs and benefits or pros and cons of any behavior.[9] The relative weighing of the pros or cons helps determine readiness for forward movement. Motivational interviewing uses this concept when it facilitates adolescents to consider the pros and cons of a given behavior to develop discrepancy between current behaviors and goals.[10]

If the perceived benefits (pros) of a behavior outweigh the perceived costs (cons), it may make no sense to consider thinking about change (ie, they will not move beyond pre-contemplation). For example, a teenager who finds that cigarettes offer the only respite she knows from a stressful home life will not be motivated to quit by being told of health risks that may affect her many years away, long after she has moved out of the challenging environment ("I'll quit then."). She will consider quitting cigarettes when she has other strategies to manage her current stress *and* she recognizes risks that affect her currently (such as high cost, reputation, yellow teeth, etc).

Because many worrisome behaviors reduce stress, it is critical that the adolescent has alternative existing positive strategies that also mitigate stress. Otherwise, the social morbidities will continue to offer present benefits that outweigh the costs. One could hypothesize that a teen would be less likely to reach toward a negative behavior in the first place (eg, using marijuana to "chill") if he already had a repertoire of effective positive strategies in place (eg, *"When I get stressed I just escape into a book."*). For this reason, time spent teaching about healthy coping can be seen both as primary and secondary prevention. In primary prevention, we reinforce a wide repertoire of activities and skill sets that serve as positive stress-reduction strategies.[11] In secondary prevention, we work with an adolescent already engaging in a negative behavior.[12] Rather than condemning his behavior, which may increase his stress, we invite him in a healing process to build positive coping strategies.

■ Coping Style

People respond to challenges differently. Researchers describe coping styles as problem-focused or emotion-focused[13] and engagement or disengagement coping.[14,15] People who use problem-focused engagement coping tend to choose 1 of 2 approaches—either they make an active effort to change the stressor itself or they change themselves enough to adapt to the stressor.[16] A major advantage of problem-focused strategies is that they either eliminate the source of the stress or help a person change enough so that the stressor has less of an effect. People who use emotion-focused disengagement coping focus on the emotions and discomfort the problem generates. People who disengage from problems can do so passively (eg, withdrawal) or actively (eg, alcohol).

Research has explored the relative benefits of problem-focused versus emotion-focused strategies.[16–19] Those who use problem-focused coping strategies tend to fare better than those who use emotion-focused coping because, if only emotions are addressed, the problem remains unresolved and can resurface. Nevertheless, emotion-focused strategies often involve seeking support from others, thereby allowing people to forge supportive connections. There is agreement that people who engage problems (via problem- or emotion-focused strategies) do better than those who disengage from problems altogether. However, disengagement may also be adaptive. Avoidance allows a person to choose the timing of when to confront an issue. It might be wise to delay a response to a problem until safety is ensured, skills are developed, and strategies are formed. Further, although we might assume disengagement strategies are unhealthy (substance use, running away), there are also healthy disengagement strategies (reading a book, working on a hobby).

■ Deriving a Comprehensive Coping Plan for Adolescents

A comprehensive stress-reduction plan should include a wide array of strategies that would prepare youth to
- Accurately assess the stressor.
- Effectively problem-solve.
- Maintain a state of health optimal for managing stress.
- Manage emotions in a healthy way.
- Use safe, healthy strategies to avoid other problems.

A stress-management plan needs to be presented quite differently for different ages both because coping strategies change across the life span[20] and because children's cognitive capacity to implement a plan varies substantially by developmental stage.[21]
- **Children.** They should be offered opportunities to learn how to feel emotionally healthy and physically strong. They will learn that they feel better after exercise and happier after they have expressed themselves creatively. Blowing bubbles can teach them about controlled and relaxing breathing. Even the youngest child can learn how much better it feels to talk if she is consistently offered a lap and a listening ear. She can learn about escape (healthy disengagement) through play, fantasy, and reading.

- **Preadolescents and early adolescents** will listen attentively as they are taught stress-reduction strategies. They will appreciate parental guidance and an acknowledgment that their lives are becoming more complex. They should be offered opportunities to practice what they have learned.
- **Mid- and late adolescents** likely will not want to hear about stress reduction from parents but may still be responsive to professionals. They can learn from written or Web-based materials and should be given opportunities to design their own plans.

All children and adolescents will learn from what their parents model. This offers a real opportunity to talk to parents about the importance of self-care. Many parents that will normally reject taking the steps to care for themselves will consider action when they are reminded how closely their children and adolescents are watching them.

■ A Stress Reduction Plan for Children and Teens

(The following plan is published in full by the American Academy of Pediatrics in *Building Resilience in Children and Teens: Giving Kids Roots and Wings*.[22])

First, it is important that young people learn to assess the stressor as a first step of coping. Then, the plan includes problem-focused engagement strategies, emotion-focused engagement strategies, and healthy disengagement strategies. It also includes basic wellness strategies that build a strong body capable of enduring stress (exercise, relaxation, nutrition, and proper sleep).

The plan has 4 broad categories and 10 points. It is not a 10-step plan; there is no designated order to approach stress. Rather, it offers a repertoire to draw from at appropriate times. For example, some strategies are cognitively based, making them unhelpful at times of severe stress. During extremely stressful moments, it may make more sense to exercise to use the stress hormones before attempting to thoughtfully resolve an issue.

Each of the points includes a variety of activities and actions to handle stress. No one should expect to use all of the techniques. Rather, they should pick an item or 2 from each point to see which best meets their needs, while remembering that the most suitable strategies change with circumstances and over time.

The stress-reduction plan includes 4 categories.

1. Tackling the problem
2. Taking care of my body
3. Dealing with emotions
4. Making the world better

Category 1: Tackling the Problem

- ***Point 1: Identify and then address the problem.*** (This point offers problem-focused engagement strategies.) Action that addresses the problem diminishes the source of stress. A key to using this strategy is to clarify the problem and then divide it into smaller pieces, committing to work on only one piece at a time. This decreases the sense of being overwhelmed and increases efficacy. Strategies to implement this point include making lists and timelines followed by a plan to address each component of the problem. Metaphorically, this is about helping teens revisualize problems from being mountains too high to be scaled into hills situated on top of each other. As they stand atop each hill, the summit appears more attainable. ▶ 8.2.1

    Strategies can be used in counseling to help teens approach larger crises or emotional issues by breaking them into manageable steps. For an example of strategies, see the "Ladder Diagram" in video 13.0, the "Tupperware Box" in video 8.13, and the "Decision Tree" in video 12.2. ▶ 8.13, 12.2, 13.0

- *Point 2: Avoid stress when possible.* (This point is a problem-focused strategy that leads to thoughtful disengagement.) This avoidance strategy teaches all young people to consider their triggers to stress and to realize that some of them can be avoided entirely. It teaches that avoiding trouble is an act of strength. A central theme of addictions treatment is to avoid the triggers that perpetuate cigarette smoking or drug use. For example, thoughtfully avoiding people, places, and things that set off stress can open the door to healthier ways of coping. This strategy should not be reserved for people in recovery and can be taught on a preventive basis. **8.2.2**

- *Point 3: Let some things go.* (This is another thoughtful, problem-focused, disengagement strategy.) While it can be useful to try to fix some problems, people who waste energy worrying about things they can't change don't have enough energy conserved to address problems they can fix. The serenity prayer, a mainstay of recovery programs, summarizes this point:

    "Grant me the serenity to accept the things I cannot change; the courage to change the things I can; and the wisdom to know the difference." **8.2.3**

Category 2: Taking Care of My Body: **7.0**

- *Point 4: The power of exercise.* Exercise may be the single most important part of the plan, and it is certainly the starting point for someone whose stress hormones prevent them from addressing any other problem or having insight into how to address a problem. When a stressed person does not exercise, their body is left feeling as if they haven't run from the "tiger." Therefore, their body senses it is still lurking and they remain hypervigilant (nervous) and their chronic stress hormones keep their blood pressure raised in preparation for the need to leap at any moment. It is not surprising, therefore, that exercise is so tightly linked to increased health and has been shown to contribute to emotional well-being and to positively affect stress, anxiety, depression, and attention-deficit/hyperactivity disorder.[23] Young people can be taught

    — *"When you are stressed, your body is saying, 'Run!' So do it."*

    — *"You may think you don't have time to exercise when you are most stressed, but that is exactly when you need it the most."*

    — *"You will be able to think better after you have used up those stress hormones."* **8.3.1**

- *Point 5: Active relaxation.* Because the parasympathetic (relaxed) and sympathetic (emergency/stressed) systems do not operate simultaneously, a key to relaxation is to stimulate the parasympathetic system. Deep methodical breathing, therefore, is the portal to relaxation. This is a mainstay of Eastern medicine techniques, yoga, and meditation, and it is even used to gain focus in the martial arts. Young people can be taught

    — *"You can flip the switch from being stressed to relaxed if you know how to turn on the relaxed system."* One technique is 4 to 8 breathing: *"Breathe deeply and slowly. Try to take a full breath. First, fill your stomach and then your chest while counting to 4. Hold that breath as long as it feels comfortable, let the breath out while counting to 8. This requires your full concentration. If your mind wanders, as it will, remind yourself to refocus on your counting and breathing. Over time, your mind will be more able to stay focused on how you are feeling now rather than past or future worries."*

    Mindfulness is a powerful technique that achieves a state of relaxation by living fully in the present while actively reminding you to let go of worries from the past and fears of the future (see Chapter 9). **8.3.2**

- **Point 6: Eat well.** Proper nutrition is essential to a healthy body and clear mind (see Chapter 7). Young people can be taught
    — *"Everyone knows good nutrition makes you healthier. Only some people realize that it also keeps you alert through the day and your mood steady. People who eat mostly junk food have highs and lows in their energy level, which harms their ability to reduce stress. Eating more fruits, vegetables, and whole grains can keep you focused for a longer time."* ▶ **8.3.3, 8.14**

- **Point 7: Sleep well.** Proper sleep is key to stress management. Some people do not sleep well because of poor sleep hygiene, including having too much stimulation in their bedrooms and keeping irregular hours. Another source of lost sleep is stress itself; people use the bed as a place to resolve their problems. The basics of sleep hygiene include
    — *"Go to sleep about the same time every night."*
    — *"Exercise 4 to 6 hours before bedtime. Your body falls asleep most easily when it has cooled down. If you exercise right before bed, you will be overheated and won't sleep well."*
    — *"A hot shower 1 hour before bedtime also helps your body relax to fall asleep."*
    — *"About half of an hour before bed, go somewhere other than your bed and do something to set your worries aside (see Point 9). Do this in dim light. If you are the kind of person who thinks about all the stuff you have to do tomorrow, make a list before you go to bed and set it aside (see Point 1). If you wake up in the middle of the night thinking, move to another spot to do your worrying. You'll get tired soon, then go back to bed."*
    — *"If you have trouble falling asleep, try 4 to 8 meditative breathing."* ▶ **8.3.4**

Category 3: Dealing With Emotions

- **Point 8: Take instant vacations.** (This point offers healthy disengagement strategies.) Sometimes the best way to de-stress is to take your mind away to a more relaxing place. Young people can be taught to take advantage of their imagination and ability to focus on other interests. Young people can be reminded to take breaks from stress.
    — **Visualization:** *"Have a favorite place where you can imagine yourself relaxing."*
    — **Enjoy your interests or hobby:** *"Get into whatever you enjoy doing that is fun and creative."* (This might include playing an instrument, drawing or writing—activities that focus and use a more creative part of a young person's brain.)
    — **Change your venue:** *"Take a walk outside."*
    — **Read:** *"Read a good book, even one you have read before."* (It may be that reading is the best diversion because it uses all of the senses—one has to imagine the sounds, sights, and smells and one also feels the emotions; there is little room left for your own worries. You are on a real vacation.)
    — **Music:** *"Listening to music can be a great break from stress and it can "reset" your emotions."* ▶ **8.4.1**

- **Point 9: Release emotional tension.** (This point offers emotion-focused engagement strategies.) A person needs to be able to express emotions rather than letting them build inside. The ideas in this category include connecting to others and letting go of feelings with verbal, written, nonverbal, and creative expression. There are a wide variety of options available to meet someone's temperament and talents.
    — **Talking to someone who is worthy of your trust:** *"Talking to a good friend, parent, teacher, or a professional, like a doctor, nurse, or counselor, can really help you get worries off your mind. Find an adult who will listen and whom you can ask for advice."*
    — **Creativity:** *"Things like art, music, poetry, singing, dance, and rap are powerful ways to let your feelings out."*
    — **Journaling:** *"Write it out!"*

— **Prayer or meditation:** *"Some people find that praying or meditation alone or with family or friends can ease their problems."*

— **Crying or laughing:** *"Some people feel so much better inside after they cry hard or laugh hard by themselves or with other people."* **8.4.2**

Category 4: Helping a Little Can Make Your World Better and Help You Feel Better

• ***Point 10: Contribute.*** Children and adolescents who consider how to serve their family, community, school, and nation will feel good about themselves, have a sense of purpose, and benefit from making a difference in other people's lives. First, they will learn that it feels good to serve, and that may reduce their sense of shame or stigma when they need to reach out for help themselves. Second, children and adolescents who serve others become surrounded by gratitude, and that can be a powerful reinforcement to continued positive behaviors. It is particularly important to adolescents who often are recipients of low expectations. Finally, people who serve others may be better able to put their own problems in perspective. **8.5**

■ Final Thoughts

We cannot take away all exposure to risk. We can, however, acknowledge that much of risk represents a young person's attempt to deal with uncomfortable feelings. Most importantly, we can make sure that young people possess a wide repertoire of positive coping strategies. When they do, the path of least resistance, during stressful times, may be the one that leads to healthy, adaptive behaviors.

•• Group Learning and Discussion ••

Healthy stress-management strategies represent both primary and secondary prevention. Primary prevention offers children and teens the tools and strategies to manage stress on a purely preventive basis to promote general wellness. In secondary prevention, these strategies offer an opportunity to shift from telling a young person what not to do toward guiding her in what she can do to both relieve stress and be healthier. The first step is to recognize that existing worrisome behaviors fill a need. In some cases, you can elicit that from young people. In other cases, they are not able to safely arrive at this insight. It is reasonable to simply ask, *"Tell me what _____ does for you."* Then, rather than condemning youths' actions, we invite them to consider healthy alternatives. Recognizing they are the experts on their own lives, it is critical to explore what already works and invite them to consider what other strategies might also work.

Break into pairs, and practice shifting young people toward healthier coping strategies. (Assume that your earlier assessment leaves you concerned, but that you have no worries of imminent self-harm.)

- A 16-year-old boy, Tony, smokes marijuana 2 to 3 times a day. His father is in prison and his mother works a double shift every day. He used to be on the track team, but now does not have time because he cares for his 3 younger siblings.
- A mother brings in her 14-year-old son, Travis, because she can't get him off of the computer. He is gaming until the early morning each night. His grades are dropping. His father is an airman who is deployed overseas. He draws cartoons for fun.
- A 15-year-old girl, Jade, is brought in by her father to discuss "laziness." She used to do well in school and now tells you that she just doesn't care anymore. She has a term paper due in 2 weeks in what used to be her favorite subject. She has had 3 months to get started. She tells you the subject is "lame." (Hint: See Point 1.)
- Lydia is a 17-year-old girl who is a straight A student. She only sleeps about 5 to 6 hours per night, because she studies until 1:00 am nightly to maintain her GPA. She plans on attending an Ivy League university. You notice that her fingernails are bitten and that she has a spot of very thin hair on her left temple. She is a wonderful writer, but stopped writing for pleasure because she has no time.

▪ References

1. Masten A. Ordinary magic: resilience processes in development. *Am Psychol.* 2001;56:227–238
2. Wills TA, Shiffman S. Coping and substance abuse: a conceptual framework. In: Shiffman S, Wills TA, eds. *Coping and Substance Use.* Orlando, FL: Academic Press; 1985
3. Brunwasser SM, Gillham JE, Kim ES. A meta-analytic review of the Penn Resiliency Program's effect on depressive symptoms. *J Consult Clin Psychol.* 2009;77(6):1042–1054
4. Reivich K, Shatté A. *The Resilience Factor.* New York, NY: Broadway Books; 2002
5. Abrahamson LY, Seligman M, Teasdale M. Learned helplessness in humans: critique and reformulation. *J Abnorm Psychol.* 1978;87:49–74
6. Beck AT. *Cognitive Therapy and the Emotional Disorders.* New York, NY: Penguin Books; 1976
7. Ellis A. *Reason and Emotion in Psychotherapy.* Carol Publishing Group; 1962
8. Prochaska JO. Decision making in the transtheoretical model of behavior change. *Med Decis Making.* 2008;28(6):845–849
9. Velicer WF, Prochaska JO, Fava JL, et al. Smoking cessation and stress management: applications of the transtheoretical model of behavior change. *Homeost.* 1998;38:216–233

10. Miller WR, Rollnick S. *Motivational Interviewing: Preparing People to Change Addictive Behavior.* New York, NY: Guilford;1991:191–202

11. Prochaska JO, Velicer WF, Rossi JS, et al. Stages of change and decisional balance for problem behaviors. *Health Psychol.* 1994;13:39–46

12. Brady SS, Tschann JM, Pasch LA, et al. Cognitive coping moderates the association between violent victimization by peers and substance use among adolescents. *J Pediatr Psychol.* 2008;34(3):304–310

13. Lazarus RS, Folkman S. *Stress, Appraisal, and Coping.* New York, NY: Springer; 1984

14. Ebata A, Moos R. Coping and adjustment in distressed and healthy adolescents. *J Appl Dev Psychol.* 1991;12:33–54

15. Tobin DL, Holroyd KA, Reynolds RV, Wigal JK. The hierarchical factor structure of the coping strategies inventory. *Cognit Ther Res.* 1989;13:343–361

16. Compas BE, Connor-Smith JK, Saltzman H, et al. Coping with stress during childhood and adolescence: problems, progress and potential in theory and research. *Psychol Bull.* 2001;127:87–127

17. Hampel P, Petermann F. Perceived stress, coping, and adjustment in adolescents. *J Adolesc Health.* 2006;38(4):409–415

18. Clark AT. Coping with interpersonal stress and psychosocial health among children and adolescents: a meta-analysis. *J Youth Adolesc.* 2006;35(1):11–24

19. Fields L, Prinz R. Coping and adjustment during childhood and adolescence. *Clin Psychol Rev.*1997;17(8):937–976

20. Diehl M, Coyle N, Labouvie-Vief G. Age and sex differences in strategies of coping and defense across the life span. *Psychol Aging.* 1996;11(1):127–139

21. Compas BE, Worsham NL, Ey S. Conceptual and developmental issues in children's coping with stress. In: La Greca AM, et al. eds. *Stress and Coping in Child Health.* New York, NY: Guilford Press; 1992

22. Ginsburg KR, Jablow MM. *Building Resilience in Children and Teens: Giving Kids Roots and Wings.* 2nd ed. Elk Grove Village, IL: American Academy of Pediatrics; 2011

23. Ratey JJ, Hagerman E. *Spark: The Revolutionary New Science of Exercise and the Brain.* New York, NY: Little, Brown and Company; 2008

■ Related Video Content

8.0 Stress Management and Coping. Ginsburg.

8.1 Stress Management and Coping/Introduction. Ginsburg.

8.2 Stress Management and Coping/Section 1/Tackling the Problem. Ginsburg.

8.2.1 Stress Management and Coping/Section 1/Tackling the Problem/Point 1: Identify and Then Address the Problem. Ginsburg.

8.2.2 Stress Management and Coping/Section 1/Tackling the Problem/Point 2: Avoid Stress When Possible. Ginsburg.

8.2.3 Stress Management and Coping/Section 1/Tackling the Problem/Point 3: Let Some Things Go. Ginsburg.

8.3 Stress Management and Coping/Section 2/Taking Care of My Body. Ginsburg.

8.3.1 Stress Management and Coping/Section 2/Taking Care of My Body/Point 4: The Power of Exercise. Ginsburg.

8.3.2 Stress Management and Coping/Section 2/Taking Care of My Body/Point 5: Active Relaxation. Ginsburg.

8.3.3 Stress Management and Coping/Section 2/Taking Care of My Body/Point 6: Eat Well. Ginsburg.

8.3.4 Stress Management and Coping/Section 2/Taking Care of My Body/Point 7: Sleep Well. Ginsburg.

■ Related Handout/Supplementary Material

Just for Teens: A Personal Plan for Managing Stress

CHAPTER 9

Mindfulness Practice for Resilience and Managing Stress and Pain

Dzung X. Vo, MD, FAAP

 Related Video Content

9.0 Mindfulness in Practice

■ Why This Matters

Mindfulness simply means, "paying attention in a particular way: on purpose, in the present moment, and nonjudgmentally".[1] Clinical mindfulness-based interventions train participants in formal and informal meditation skills to promote coping and resilience. Mindfulness-based interventions are emerging as a feasible and effective method to promote resilience and coping among adolescents with chronic stress, mood symptoms, chronic illness, and pain. **9.8**

> ●● **Much of our stress and suffering comes from being pulled away from the present moment. Our minds may be caught in regrets about the past, worries about the future, or judgments about the present. Mindfulness is practiced with a sense of loving-kindness, being fully present with whatever is inside and around you in the present moment, and meeting it with kindness and without judgment. ●●**

■ Case: 17-Year-Old Female With Back Pain

Susan is a 17-year-old female who suffered a serious injury several years ago. Since that time, she has suffered from severe, chronic back pain. The pain profoundly disrupted her functioning at school and at home, and significantly impacted her stress and mood. Susan had seen multiple medical and surgical specialists over several years, and had not experienced significant relief with standard therapies. She was beginning to lose hope, feeling, *"I can't have a future"* and *"This will never get better."*

Through the course of our initial discussions, Susan was able to identify relationships between her mind state and her body state, observing that when she was feeling stressed and depressed, her back pain worsened and was more difficult to cope with, and vice versa (her back pain worsened her stress and mood). I verbally reinforced this insight, and used this strength as a starting point to discuss the potential role of mindfulness training as a mind-body intervention to help her cope with pain and improve her functioning and her quality of life. Susan agreed to try an 8-week individual mindfulness training program, adapted from mindfulness-based stress reduction (MBSR).

Together with Susan's mother, every week we learned and practiced formal mindfulness practices such as sitting meditation and body scan meditation, as well as informal mindfulness practices such as eating meditation and walking meditation. We discussed and explored Susan's experiences, successes, and challenges with mindfulness practice at home. Ultimately, I encouraged Susan to develop her capacity, as much as possible, to be mindful in every moment and every activity of her everyday life, training herself to continually bring awareness to the present moment without judgment, and with kindness and compassion.

After 8 weeks of mindfulness training and practice, Susan reported that her pain had improved somewhat but, more importantly, her relationship with her pain and with her body had transformed profoundly. *"I'm fine with having the pain now…as opposed to learning how to ignore my pain, I've learned how to accept my pain. What makes me really happy is not being stressed about the pain."* Susan's mother agreed with her observations, and, as a side benefit, reported that the whole family benefited from the mindfulness training. Susan's newfound sense of hope helped her to complete high school, and she is now planning to enter the health care field.

■ Mindfulness: Background

Mindfulness practice has its historic origins in Eastern meditation and traditions, and can also be found in wisdom traditions worldwide. Jon Kabat-Zinn and others[2,3] have developed secular (nonreligious) mindfulness-based training programs such as MBSR, adapting mindfulness practices for application in clinical and community settings. Other evidence-based mindfulness-based interventions include mindfulness-based cognitive therapy for depression, mindfulness-based relapse prevention for substance abuse, and mindfulness-based childbirth and parenting.

A large body of literature in adult populations demonstrates benefits of mindfulness-based clinical interventions in heterogeneous disorders and populations, including chronic pain, mood disorders, substance abuse, and coping with chronic illness.[4] Recent studies suggest that mindfulness training may alter physiological parameters, including immune function, brain gray matter concentrations visible on magnetic resonance imaging scans, and even cellular telomeres associated with aging.[5-7]

Mindfulness-based interventions are now being developed and offered to children and youth in medical and mental health settings, as well as schools, community-based settings, and juvenile justice settings. Research on mindfulness with youth is in its infancy and is developing rapidly. Early studies on mindfulness with youth show promise for potential improvements in emotional regulation, attention, learning, and mental health symptoms.[8,9]

Mindfulness practice is based on the observation that much of our stress and suffering comes from being pulled away from the present moment. We spend much of our time in "autopilot" mode, going through the motions of life without being fully present in the here and now. Our body may be in one place, and our mind may be somewhere else entirely. Often our minds may be caught in regrets about the past, worries about the future, or judgments about the present. In this ruminative or "mindless" state, we are vulnerable to "reacting" to stressful and painful situations from a state of fear, with our higher cortical brain function (our prefrontal cortex, or "human brain") overwhelmed by the fight, flight, or freeze stress response (sometimes described as the "reptile brain"). We may lose regulation and integration of our brain and emotions, and get caught in negative mood states and/or reactive behaviors that can make the situation worse.

Dr Daniel Siegel's "hand model of the brain" is a concrete and simple way of teaching what happens in our brains and bodies, when we become overwhelmed with stress and "lose it."[10] Children as young as 5 years can understand the hand model of the brain. Fortunately, we can learn how to reengage the "human" part of our brain using mindfulness and other practices, thereby reestablishing integration and healthy regulation. From this state of present-moment awareness, we can see and respond to situations with more wisdom and clarity, and access our innate capacity for healing.

8.6

For example, in the case study, Susan's chronic pain led to recurrent thoughts like, *"I wish that injury had never happened," "My pain is always terrible and will never get better,"* and *"I won't be able to have a future."* Every time she experienced physical pain, these thoughts were repeatedly reinforced, which, in turn, amplified the suffering caused by her physical sensations. The thoughts pulled her away from her actual present moment experiences. She became caught in ruminative judgments, regrets, and worries, which triggered and reinforced her stress response in a vicious cycle. Mindfulness training helped Susan to free herself from this cycle, and change her relationship with her thoughts, emotions, and physical sensations. Susan rediscovered and strengthened her capacity to be awake to the present moment, deeply in touch with what was happening in the here and now, with an open heart and without judging. All youth have this innate capacity, and systematic mindfulness training helps them to employ this capacity more consistently and effectively.

Adolescence is a particularly critical window both to the vulnerability to stress and the opportunity for intervention to promote stress management and resilience. Adults expect adolescents to be able to regulate their emotions, manage stress, plan for the future, act with empathy and compassion, and think abstractly. However, adolescent brains do not fully mature until the mid-20s, especially in the prefrontal areas responsible for executive functioning, integration, and regulation. Mindfulness practice is a concrete tool to stimulate and promote neural circuits associated with resilience and emotional regulation, and may promote healthier adolescent brain development.[10] Teaching mindfulness to youth has the potential to help them develop lifelong coping habits and profoundly affect their life trajectory.

■ Here's How It Works: Office-Based Mindfulness Training

- **Step 1: Psychoeducation on brain, body, stress, and coping.** Provide background on stress, mind, body, and coping (see chapters 7 and 8). The key messages are
  — Everyone has stress and pain. Stress is inevitable. Suffering may be, at least to some degree, optional. What matters is how you manage stress and pain.
  — You can cope with stress and pain in a positive (healthy) or negative (unhealthy) direction. (This message should avoid the implication of judgment.)
  — Symptoms of stress and pain can be experienced in both the body and the mind, and the body and mind are interconnected in complex ways. Practices that integrate the mind and body can promote health and resilience.
  — Consider teaching teens and families the "hand model of the brain" to illustrate what happens under stress.
  — You can learn tools to engage your whole brain and innate strength to manage stress and pain in a healthy way.
- **Step 2: Setting the stage for mindfulness.** Adapt the information in the text above to offer a definition of mindfulness and brief background on the clinical application and potential benefits of mindfulness practice. Use motivational interviewing techniques to explore and promote engagement and motivation. If the teen is somewhat open-minded

or motivated to try mindfulness, then set the stage for mindfulness training. Key messages to convey include

— Encourage an attitude of "beginner's mind": letting go of preconceived ideas, expectations, and judgments.

— Tell the teen, *"As long as you are breathing, there is more right with you than there is wrong with you."* Mindfulness is a deeply strength-based approach, based on the insight that if you can learn to allow yourself to be present with whatever you are experiencing, you will rediscover your innate strength and capacity to more skillfully handle any situation, any feeling, any emotion you might encounter. You do not need to keep running away, covering up, fighting, or denying anything.

— One of the most important "mindful qualities" is loving kindness (or compassion, friendliness, or heartfulness). When you practice mindfulness with a sense of loving-kindness, it means you are being fully present with whatever is inside you and around you in the present moment, and meeting it with kindness and without judgment.

— Another mindful quality is an attitude of curiosity: experiencing each moment with the question, *"What is happening right now?"*—just posing the question with an open heart and mind, and without necessarily trying to find or get attached to an "answer."

— Mindfulness means becoming aware of, and then letting go of, judgments about yourself. This includes judgments about whether or not you are doing mindfulness "correctly."

— Relaxation and calmness are common side effects of mindfulness practice, but relaxation is not the explicit goal of mindfulness practice. Mindfulness means to become aware of whatever you are experiencing, whether it is pleasant or unpleasant. So, in some cases, you may feel relaxed, but, in other cases, you may not. Either way is OK. The important thing is the awareness, with an attitude of kindness and curiosity.

- **Step 3: Introducing a formal mindfulness practice.** Mindfulness of breathing is a simple practice that forms the foundation of other mindfulness practices. The body scan is useful for patients with insomnia, chronic pain, and other mind-body syndromes. Formal mindfulness practices can be practiced in as little as 3 to 5 minutes, or up to 30 minutes or longer. Other mindfulness practices include walking meditation, loving-kindness meditation, and eating meditation. Formal practices can be guided by voice or by an audio recording, or self-guided (silent). Encourage the teen to set aside time in her day for a formal mindfulness practice every day (for example, in the morning or before bedtime). Remind her that short periods (even 3 to 5 minutes) of frequent practice are more likely to be beneficial than longer infrequent practices. See the handouts at the end of this chapter for details on mindfulness of breathing and body scan. Visit the Kelty Mental Health Resource Centre Web site (http://keltymentalhealth.ca/healthy-living/mindfulness) for free ▶ **9.1, 9.2** audio recordings of guided mindfulness meditations.[11]

- **Step 4: Introducing informal mindfulness practices.** Formal mindfulness practices are practices that you set aside time to do. Informal mindfulness practices, on the other hand, bring that same mindful, present-moment, and nonjudgmental awareness to all activities of daily living. Concrete mindfulness practices that can be done formally or informally are walking meditation and eating meditation. After ▶ **9.3** demonstrating and practicing an informal mindfulness practice with the teen, encourage her to use her creativity and intelligence to bring present-moment, nonjudgmental awareness to activities that she already does during the day, such as walking, eating, talking to a friend, or riding the bus. Encourage her to find and use reminders in the environment (such as phones or school bells ringing) as virtual "bells of mindfulness," reminding her to come back to the present moment, breathe 3 mindful breaths, and carry on in mindfulness. Remind her that the mindful qualities of kindness and curiosity are available in every moment, and that, by practicing coming back to the present moment over and over again, she can train herself to live life more fully and handle her stress and pain more effectively.

Office-based teaching and practice can be performed in a few repeated brief weekly office visits, and subsequently reinforced periodically. For teens who may benefit from or need more intensive mindfulness training, consider referring to a provider with expertise in mindfulness-based interventions, and/or referring to a formal group mindfulness training program (see Related Web Sites). Teens in our formal mindfulness programs often report that after 8 weeks of mindfulness training, they have learned more than just a "technique" to apply in specific situations. They have learned a new way of being and a healthier way of looking at the world, and have regained hope and courage that they thought was lost.

The most important aspect in teaching mindfulness to teens—more important than what words you say or what format or techniques you apply—is the quality of your own mindfulness practice.

■ Here's How It Works: Mindfulness for Providers

There is growing interest and literature in mindfulness training for providers as a tool to promote stress management, decrease burnout, and increase empathy and effective clinical communication skills.[12] Moreover, having a personal mind- **9.5, 9.9** fulness practice can be very useful for teaching mindfulness effectively to teens. When you teach mindfulness directly from your own experience and practice, you role-model and embody mindfulness with an authenticity that is critical to teaching this practice. If you are interested in teaching mindfulness to teens, first begin to develop your own mindfulness practice. You can start by enrolling in an 8-week MBSR course or other mindfulness training program in your local area (see Related Web Sites). Once you begin to experience mindfulness practice and its benefits for yourself, you can slowly start to teach the practices that you have found useful in your own life.

●● Group Learning and Discussion ●●

Discuss
1. Who among our youth would benefit from the practice of mindfulness?
2. How might it help us better serve youth and their families?
3. How could we make it feasible to incorporate mindfulness into our practice? Should we consider group mindfulness sessions for select youth? Should we investigate mindfulness training referral resources for our youth? Could we at least make Dr Vo's explanations available for our youth and their families?
4. How might we benefit as providers from personal mindfulness practice?

Practice
Mindfulness is far better practiced than discussed. Use the supplementary tools as well as the videos to prepare yourself to incorporate mindfulness into your practice and, perhaps, your own self-care regimen.

■ References

1. Kabat-Zinn J. *Wherever You Go, There You Are: Mindfulness Meditation in Everyday Life*. New York, NY: Hyperion; 1994
2. Kabat-Zinn, J. *Full Catastrophe Living: Using the Wisdom of Your Body and Mind to Face Stress, Pain, and Illness*. 5th ed. New York, NY: Delta; 1990
3. Stahl B, Goldstein E. *A Mindfulness-Based Stress Reduction Workbook*. Oakland, CA: New Harbinger Publications; 2010
4. Baer R. Mindfulness training as a clinical intervention: a conceptual and empirical review. *Clin Psychol Sci Pract*. 2003;10:125–143
5. Davidson RJ, Kabat-Zinn J, Schumacher J, et al. Alterations in brain and immune function produced by mindfulness meditation. *Psychosom Med*. 2003;65(4):564–570
6. Holzel BK, Carmody J, Vangel M, et al. Mindfulness practice leads to increases in regional brain gray matter density. *Psychiatry Res*. 2011;191(1):36–43
7. Jacobs TL, Epel ES, Lin J, et al. Intensive meditation training, immune cell telomerase activity, and psychological mediators. *Psychoneuroendocrinology*. 2011;36(5):664–681
8. Burke CA. Mindfulness-based approaches with children and adolescents: a preliminary review of current research in an emerging field. *J Child Fam Stud*. 2010;19:133–144
9. Harnett PH, Dawe S. Review: the contribution of mindfulness-based therapies for children and families and proposed integration. *Child Adolesc Ment Health*. 2012. DOI: 10.1111/j.1475-3588.2011.00643.x
10. Siegel, Daniel J. *Mindsight: The New Science of Personal Transformation*. New York, NY: Bantam; 2010
11. BC Children's Hospital. Kelty Mental Health Resource Centre, BC Children's Hospital. http://keltymentalhealth.ca/healthy-living/mindfulness. Accessed September 3, 2013
12. Krasner MS, et al. Association of an educational program in mindful communication with burnout, empathy, and attitudes among primary care physicians. *JAMA*. 2009;302(12):1284–1293

■ Suggested Reading

Vo DX, Park MJ. Stress and stress management among youth and young men. *Am J Mens Health*. 2008;2(4):353–366

Willard C. *Child's Mind: Mindfulness Practices to Help Our Children Become More Focused, Calm, and Relaxed*. Berkeley, CA: Parallax Press; 2010

■ Related Video Content

9.0 Mindfulness in Practice. Vo.

9.1 The Body Scan. Vo.

9.2 Awareness of Breathing. Vo.

9.3 Mindful Walking. Vo.

9.4 Getting Practical: Bringing Mindfulness Into Your Life. Vo.

9.5 Mindfulness as a Tool to Increase Your Clinical Effectiveness. Vo.

9.6 Planting the Seeds…Trusting the Flower Might Bloom. Vo.

9.7 Mindfulness as a Means to Increase Self-acceptance, Diminish Shame, and Defeat Self-hatred. Vo.

9.8 Mindfulness: Youth Voices (Kelty Mental Health Resource Centre). Vo, Youth.

9.9 Mindfulness Allows Us to Remain Fully Present Even Amidst Our Exposure to Suffering. Vo.

8.6 A Simple Explanation of How Stress Affects the Brain. Vo.

■ Related Handouts/Supplementary Materials

Sample Guided Mindfulness of Breathing Meditation

The Body Scan

■ Related Web Sites

Greater Good Guide to Mindfulness, University of California, Berkeley
http://educ.ubc.ca/research/ksr/docs/mindfulnessguide_may2010.pdf
Short articles written for non-specialist audience, on mindfulness background, mindful parenting, and teaching mindfulness in prisons, schools, and with veterans.

Kelty Mental Health Resource Centre, BC Children's Hospital
http://keltymentalhealth.ca/healthy-living/mindfulness
This Web site offers free audio recordings of guided mindfulness meditations that we use in our mindfulness for teens programs at BC Children's Hospital.

Mindfulness in Education Network
www.mindfuled.org
A network of professionals interested in mindfulness with children and youth. Resources include an e-mail listserv and professional conferences.

University of Massachusetts Center for Mindfulness in Medicine, Health Care, and Society
www.umassmed.edu/content.aspx?id=41252
Mindfulness-Based Stress Reduction (MBSR) was developed here, and this Web site offers numerous resources for clinicians, patients, and researchers.

Approaches to Reach Youth and Facilitate Positive Change

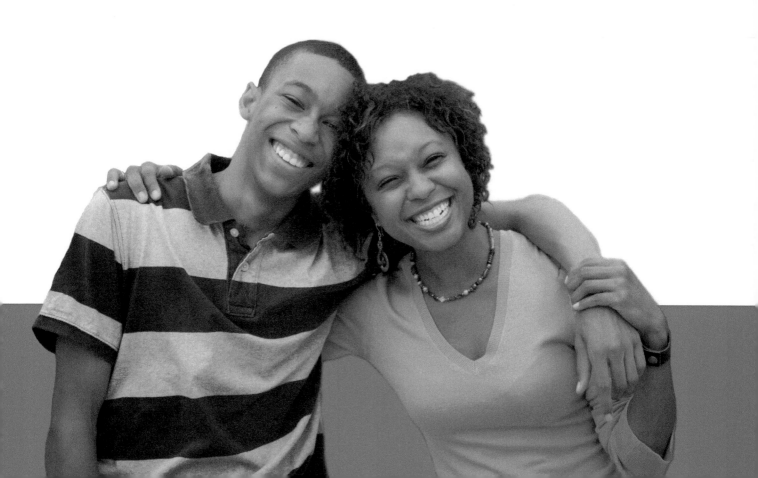

CHAPTER 10

Addressing Demoralization: Eliciting and Reflecting Strengths

Kenneth R. Ginsburg, MD, MS Ed, FAAP, FSAHM

 Related Video Content

10.0.1 An Introduction to Behavioral Change: Youth Will Not Make Positive Choices if They Don't Believe in Their Potential to Change
10.0.2 Addressing Demoralization: Eliciting and Reflecting Strengths

■ Why This Matters

A fundamental aspect of contemplating change is consideration of whether change is even possible.[1] If a person does not believe she is capable of change, she will stifle consideration of progress, or perhaps deny the existence of the problem altogether to avoid the frustration that accompanies powerlessness. It is easier to deny a problem exists than to meet with failure, especially if a person has repeated experience of having failed. For this reason, the first step toward behavioral change may be attaining confidence that one can change.

> **Young adults who have changed their life path often recall a pivotal moment when a caring professional made them realize they had potential.**

Confidence is rooted in competence.[2] A person gains confidence partially through receiving and believing feedback from others that he has demonstrated capabilities. He solidifies confidence when further actions demonstrate the experience of success.

A person's confidence is undermined when he receives and internalizes messages that he is incapable. Even typical adolescents absorb messages that they are the source of problems and prone to impulsive rather than reasoned action.[3] However, some adolescents have heard undermining messages consistently that have not been counterbalanced by supportive relationships. These youth have learned to see themselves as undeserving and have grown to see their destiny as out of their control. Still other youth have made repeated efforts to change their life circumstances and have met with failure. These latter 2 groups may become demoralized and, therefore, particularly resistant to the possibility of change. They are deserving of a strength-based approach that helps them recognize they can control their destiny. A first step toward this goal is facilitating them to recognize they possess skill sets they can use to change their life circumstances.

■ How to Combat Demoralization

A professional using a problem- or risk-focused approach may begin with a statement of the problem and offer reasons why current behaviors will cause harm or lead to a feared outcome. This approach does not recognize the context of a young person's life and may leave him thinking he is seen only as "a problem." If this occurs, it can reinforce a sense of shame, undermining both the potential for change and the forging of a therapeutic relationship. On the other hand, if after a comprehensive SSHADESS screen, which included close attention to existing strengths, you can place the problem amidst a sea of strengths, the young person is less likely to feel ashamed and more likely to be receptive to guidance. This may be even more effective if the existing strengths can be tightly linked to the desired behavior.

 10.0.1, 10.13

Several examples help to illustrate this point.

- A young person who is smoking marijuana to relieve stress, to chill, may possess tremendous sensitivity and a real desire to improve the challenges at home. He may be smoking precisely because he is the kind of person who cares deeply.
- A young woman who wants to become a mother has the desire to be nurturing.
- The 15-year-old drug dealer is also an entrepreneur who may be driven to contribute to his family.
- The gang member has a deep sense of loyalty and a desire to belong and to feel protected from a dangerous environment.

Recognizing the positive contexts that drive a negative behavior neither condones the behavior nor diminishes our desire to address it. Rather, it allows us to see youth in a way that will prevent shame from being inadvertently communicated through our interaction. The goal is to build on the point of strength and hope for a ripple effect that will diminish the teen's need to continue engaging in the maladaptive behavior. For example, a young person who uses drugs but who is also recognized for her sensitivity may be more receptive to other means to diminish stress as well as strategies to creatively and safely express sensitivity.

An approach to intervention that both recognizes strength and invites a collaborative approach follows: 10.0.2

Step 1: **Elicit.** Listen for context and strengths.

Step 2: **Reflect.** Tell the young person what you admire about her and what you see as her strengths.

Step 3: **Pause.** Take a breath for a moment and allow the youth to absorb the genuineness of your reflection. It may be a rare or singular experience for the teen to be noticed for what she is doing right.

Step 4: **Share** what you may be worried about. Ideally, tell the teen why you are concerned that the current behavior may get in the way of achieving her stated goals.

Step 5: **Ask permission** to discuss the issue further. This may be an unusual experience for the adolescent, as young people are not usually asked whether they want to engage in a conversation.

If the youth does suggest she wants to engage in further discussion, consider using motivational interviewing techniques to further increase motivation to change (see Chapter 11).

■ Case I

Lisa is a 14-year-old girl who tells her doctor that her grades have been dropping and that she is worried that they will prevent her from becoming the pediatric nurse practitioner she has dreamed of becoming. The doctor refrains from launching into a talk about the importance of good grades, and simply asks her why she thinks her grades have declined.

Lisa explains that her mother relies on her pretty heavily to take care of her 3 younger siblings. She describes how much she loves her mother and understands she is overburdened, especially because she is working extra hours to make sure she will have enough money to send everyone to college.

Lisa quickly jumps in, *"I really love taking care of my little brothers and sister!"* She helps them with homework, picks out their clothes for the next day, makes sure they take their baths, and even does bedtime prayers with them. *"They are my heart."* It's just that after she spends so much time helping them, there is very little time for her own homework, and she is worried about herself.

The doctor comments that it sounds stressful and asks her how she manages that stress. *"To chill,"* she said, she smokes marijuana, *"only after they go to bed. I never smoke in front of my brothers and sister."*

Lisa could be reprimanded or given 40 reasons not to smoke marijuana, but that would shame her and likely have no yield other than increasing her stress level, perhaps leading directly to increased marijuana use.

Instead, the doctor listened silently to her story without interruption or criticism. By listening to her intently, all that she is doing right becomes clear. When she finishes talking, the doctor says, *"We need you to be a pediatric nurse. Look how good you are with little kids. You get your brothers and sister dinner. You make sure they're safe. You bathe them and put them to bed. You're really responsible. You've already proven how good you are at caring for people and how much you love children."* After a short pause, he states, *"I'm feeling worried, though, about how much marijuana you are smoking and am concerned that may interfere with your future plans. Can we talk about this?"*

It is so much easier for young people to deal with why we are worried if we first note their successes. When we get their permission to address the problem, we get buy-in and offer them the kind of control and self-confidence they need to be willing to consider taking steps to change.

Listening and reflecting takes on even greater importance for the demoralized youth who may have little experience with a person seeing the best in them. Central to both the resilience and youth development frameworks is the notion that youth live up or down to people's expectations of them. Young people who have internalized low expectations do not always see their potential to change. For them, it may be transformative for someone to notice positive traits.

In this author's experience, it is common for older teens or young adults who have changed their life path to recall a pivotal moment when a caring professional made them realize they had potential.

For these youth, listen silently and with full attention as their story unfolds. Rather than considering your next counseling steps, allow yourself to view the youth through a different prism; think only of what you admire about the young person. Even a patient whose history concerns you deeply is being honest. Many youth with the most traumatic histories have displayed tremendous resilience. They have been survivors; doing the best they can to deal with a world that wasn't fair to them. Older teens who "have been there and done that" are often able to display great insight into their behaviors. It is common for these very same youth who have had the roughest lives thus far to ▶ 10.8 dream of becoming helping professionals so they can help other children have smoother lives.

■ Case 2

Shawn is a 17-year-old young man who has just been released from a youth detention facility after a short stay. He grew up in a highly stressed household where abuse was pervasive. He recalls witnessing his father beating his mother when he was as young as 3 years. He recalls trying to stand between them to protect his mother. His jaws clench as he tells you how his father would throw him against a wall and would reprimand him for his interference. Shawn learned not to cry because, when he did, he was told, *"Men don't cry,"* and *"You want to be a man, I'll show you how to be a man,"* as his father would proceed with the beating. His mother turned to drugs to forget about the pain and died when Shawn was 11 years old. His father has been in jail since Shawn was 12 and he was sent to live with his grandmother. When he was too "disrespectful" to her he was put into foster care. He has been through 6 placements and was maltreated in 2 of them. He turned to drugs himself and was arrested for possession when he was 15. Most recently, he was arrested for dealing, but that was found to be a case of mistaken identity.

Shawn is an artist who uses paper to release his feelings. He hasn't used drugs since he was 15 years old, except for one brief period when he was particularly stressed. He has a girlfriend who he cares about deeply and whom he would, *"never put my hands on."* He dreams of being a youth services worker who could help abused children. His eyes redden as he shares the fact that someone like him doesn't have a chance to have that dream come true, he really isn't good at school and only made it to the ninth grade.

The social worker listens and notes how bright this young man is. He notices his sincerity and his genuine desire to become a youth services worker. However, he also notes that the teen does not believe in his potential and likely lacks the confidence to take even the first steps necessary to return to get his education. He also has no support structure in place to facilitate him through the administrative steps necessary for him to follow through on his vision. In essence, he lacks the confidence and the skills to move his dreams from contemplation to action.

He retells the young man his story, perhaps in a way that the teen has never experienced previously: *"Wow. You have been through a lot. More than anyone your age deserves to have been through. I wish I could say that your story shocks me, that I've never heard anything like it before. That you were the first young man who has had to suffer through abuse and see the tragedy of your mother being hurt and turning to drugs. But the truth is that I've seen it too often. But you know what? Most of those kids are seething with anger. I know you've been there and that's probably why you acted out earlier. Many of those kids turn to drugs themselves to deal with the pain. I know you've "been there, done that" for a little while too, but you figured out on your own to stop. Instead, you turned to art to deal with your feelings rather than just letting them cloud over. Many of those kids take out their anger on women, but you know how to care for women. Many of those kids have given up hope and just dwell in anger, but you want to help kids. You want to take your experience and make the world better. Teach me about you. Teach me about how despite all that you've been through, you've come out as a caring man committed to protecting children."*

After a brief discussion where the young person becomes emotional and shares his insights, the social worker continues one step at a time allowing the teen to determine his readiness for each option: *"You deserve to have your dreams come true. Many children will benefit from your experience. You also deserve healing first, to help you get past some of the pain that happened to you. Do you have any ideas about what will work for you? May I suggest some healthy ways that help people cope? (See Chapter 8.) You are so good at talking. May I arrange for you to have your own counselor who will listen to you, and perhaps guide you as you take next steps? Does now feel like the right time to think about getting the education you need? If so, I would love to connect you to a community resource that helps young people return to school. Can we schedule a check-in for 2 weeks from today to follow the progress you've made?"*

•• Group Learning and Discussion ••

It is so easy to see risk. It is much harder to look beneath the surface to see strengths, yet it is key to positioning you as a change agent. It is an active choice to decide to see youth through a positive prism, and it may take practice before it comes routinely. It begins with a SSHADESS screen that starts with teens describing their positive attributes. Then, it is about listening for strength. For example, it may involve allowing yourself to be surprised by the compassion some people possess despite the fact they were offered little. It may be respecting the resilience they demonstrate. It may be admiring their plans to repair the world, so that it looks more like they wished it had looked for them.

Exercise

(1) Share stories about some of the youth who you have cared for who maintained a positive outlook despite dire circumstances. (2) Practice the eliciting and reflecting approach in pairs, with one of you taking on the role of professional and the other that of the youth.

Ongoing Practice

Make a point of sharing inspirational stories within your practice. Share especially those stories of youth that surprise you. This will lead to different expectations for all youth.

- Especially when you are struggling to find the positive in a young person, debrief with a colleague whose role will be to elicit the strengths the youth may be exhibiting in that situation.
- Share with each other how the tone and demeanor of your interactions with demoralized youth changes when using this strength-based approach.
- Share with each other how the experience of seeing marginalized youth through a positive lens changes your work experience, and why it may diminish your likelihood of burnout.

■ References

1. Prochaska JO. Decision making in the transtheoretical model of behavior change. *Med Decis Mak.* 2008;28(6):845–849
2. Schwarzer R, Fuchs R. Changing risk behaviors and adopting health behaviors: the role of self-efficacy beliefs. In: Bandura A, ed. *Self-efficacy in Changing Societies.* Cambridge, United Kingdom: Cambridge University Press; 1997
3. Hein K. Framing and reframing. *J Adolesc Health.* 1997;21:214–217

■ Related Video Content

10.0.1 An Introduction to Behavioral Change: Youth Will Not Make Positive Choices if They Don't Believe in Their Potential to Change. Ginsburg.

10.0.2 Addressing Demoralization: Eliciting and Reflecting Strengths. Ginsburg.

10.1 Covenant House Staff Share How Recognizing Strengths Positions Them to Support Progress. Covenant House PA.

10.2 YouthBuild Staff Share How Recognizing Strengths Positions Them to Support Progress. YouthBuild Philadelphia.

■ Related Handout/Supplementary Material

The SSHADESS Screen

CHAPTER 11

Motivational Interviewing

Nimi Singh, MD, MPH, MA

 Related Video Content

11.0 Motivational Interviewing With Adolescents

■ Why This Matters

Adolescents' health and well-being are tightly linked to the behavioral choices they make. These choices, although made in the teen years, can have a lifelong impact. Therefore, it is imperative that youth-serving professionals become adept at supporting adolescents in choosing to adopt healthier lifestyle behaviors. Motivational interviewing (MI) has been shown to be an effective counseling style that promotes healthy behavioral change, both in adults and in adolescents.

> Motivational interviewing is an empathetic, person-centered counseling style. It is based on the recognition that the most powerful motivations for changing our behaviors don't come from others, but from us.

■ What Is Motivational Interviewing?

Motivational interviewing is more than a set of techniques. It is an empathetic, person-centered counseling style. It is based on the recognition that the most powerful motivations for changing our behaviors don't come from others, but from ourselves. This approach creates the conditions for positive behavioral change by gently guiding youth into articulating their own reasons for change, and identifying how they hope to achieve it. It is well-suited for brief clinical encounters; evidenced-based (>200 clinical trials in both adults and adolescents); grounded in health behavior theory; verifiable and generalizable; and can be delivered by a wide range of professionals who are addressing a variety of behaviors.

Motivational interviewing is based on 2 assumptions. First, a person's motivation to change his or her behavior can be elicited by a conversation with someone skilled to draw out the person's own reasons for changing. Simply telling someone why they need to change is experienced as confrontational and, as such almost always creates resistance to the suggestion. Alternately, empathy, understanding, and exploration of the young person's experience creates a space for self-reflection and the desire for change. The second assumption is that ambivalence toward the possibility of change is normal and to be expected. In contemplating a change, there are always competing positive and negative feelings, a weighing of pros and cons.

What is unique in MI is that it is the *youth* who articulates arguments for change and the treatment plan. The role of the professional is *not* to provide reasons for behavior change, but rather to act as a facilitator, guiding the adolescent through questions and reflections, listening for ambivalence in the teen's own words, and reflecting back negative and positive aspects of both the current behavior and of the desired behavior change. The professional also needs to be able to support self-efficacy (that is, the confidence that one can achieve what one sets out to do). This is done by pointing out strengths and previous successes, and acknowledging the difficulties of making the behavioral change. The practitioner also needs to, above all, avoid resistance by refraining from lecturing and arguing with the adolescent. Finally, the practitioner asks teens what *they* want to do/are willing to do; their answers often become the starting point or goal for the treatment plan.

■ Underlying Theoretical Framework: Stages of Change

Prochaska and DiClemente[1] articulated the stages of change model, in which they hypothesized that behavioral change doesn't happen in one stage, but rather that a person goes through several stages before adopting and maintaining a new behavior. These stages are (1) pre-contemplation, (2) contemplation, (3) action, (4) maintenance, and (5) relapse. Pre-contemplation means that the person isn't even thinking about changing her behavior, and if asked if they were considering it, they would say "no." Contemplation is the stage where the person is waxing and waning toward the idea of change, and wrestling with the reasons for and against changing their behavior or habit. This is the stage of ambivalence. The action stage occurs when ambivalence is subsiding, and the person is ready and motivated to implement the change. Maintenance is the stage when the person continues to exert effort to continue the new behavior. Of note, this stage is also often the time when services and support are withdrawn. This is highly unfortunate because this stage is an especially vulnerable time, and life stressors may cause the person to relapse back into the old behavior. For this reason, it is critical to have frequent follow-up to reinforce the benefits of the changes while youth are in the "maintenance" stage. Relapse represents a return to the previous behavior, is common, and should be expected for most long-term behavioral changes.

Ideally, we hope to avoid relapse, but, if it occurs, it is critical to support return to the desired behavior afterward. Once there has been a lapse or relapse, the individual reenters the process at either pre-contemplation (becoming discouraged or convinced that they can't change after all), contemplation (begins the weighing of pros and cons again), or action (jumps back on track and picks up the new behavior once again with little hesitation). One of the most important points to remember is that it is the professional who plays a *key* role in influencing a person's reentry point into the process! Youth will experience guilt and shame even when there is no one blaming them. This often causes an adolescent to be defensive from the get-go. It is critical, therefore, for the professional to shift the conversation from "relapse" to "success": this is done by focusing on the period prior to the relapse as a success and asking how that success was possible for that long. Then have the young person identify what stressor triggered the relapse. Following this, have her brainstorm what would help avoid a future relapse, should the stressors recur. We will give an example of this later in the chapter.

When first articulated by Prochaska and DiClemente,[1] a stage between contemplation and action was termed preparation. For the purposes of this discussion, preparation is incorporated into the contemplation stage. Here, the pros and cons of behavior change are explored, and potential supports and barriers are identified and addressed, in order to prepare the individual for taking action.

■ Rethinking Conventional Training

Why doesn't our conventional training work optimally in counseling youth? Most of us were trained in a directive counseling style that looks (or at least feels) something like the following admittedly simplified approach:

I'll ask you close-ended questions.

I'll tell you what's wrong with you.

I'll tell you what you need to do.

I'll assume that you're going to do it.

This approach is often adequate for simple, short-term behaviors and interventions, such as taking a medication for a short time. This approach also works well for motivated youth/families (those in the action stage).

Motivational interviewing, alternatively, is a combination of 3 counseling styles: (1) following (establish rapport, have youth expand story), (2) guiding (asking questions that support self-reflection), and (3) gently directing (asking permission before giving information first, checking in after). These styles rely heavily on open-ended questions, reflecting back what a teen says, and waiting for further elaboration before offering information. This approach works well for youth ambivalent about behavioral change (in contemplation stage).

We like working with young people in the action stage because our conventional tools fit well with their stage of change; they cooperate and typically do what we suggest; we tend not to experience anger, frustration, and impatience; and they make us feel competent. We may not like working with youth in the contemplation (ambivalence) stage because our tools *don't* fit with their stage of change, and they don't do what we suggest. We then experience anger and frustration when we see them again, and may even feel relief when they don't show up. We "pathologize" ambivalence when it's, in fact, the norm when it comes to behavioral change. In the end, we may become disheartened and give up on the youth we serve (and ourselves), saying:

"I can't help someone who doesn't want to be helped."

"I can't help someone who doesn't admit to having a problem."

We don't realize we're inadvertently perpetuating the resistance.

■ Who Are the Youth We See?

Studies estimate that, in the case of health care, only 30% of patients who present to clinic are actually in action stage! This means that a full 70% are in pre-contemplation or contemplation stages. We, therefore, *over*estimate the motivation of those who say they're ready to change (we give them information without exploring possible ambivalence/barriers to change). At the same time, we *under*estimate the motivation of those who indicate no interest in change. We don't realize that reluctance is often due to underlying values, beliefs, and fears associated with changing the behavior. When we understand these, we can help reconnect adolescents to their own values, and help them see how certain behaviors are incongruent with what they care about the most in their lives. In other words, MI may be *the* treatment of choice for ambivalence to change for roughly 70% of our population!

■ Philosophical Approach

The approach to the adolescent, instead of simply imparting information, is exploratory. It is respectful, nonjudgmental, reflective, and compassionate. We are asked to shift our goal from "fixing it" to "listening for understanding." In doing so, we are then able to create the environment in which "change talk" can be elicited.

■ Principles

The foundation for successful implementation of MI is based on the following guiding principles:

1. Establish rapport, and meet youth where they are. A very effective way to achieve this is to start with a broad psychosocial interview.

   "How are things going? What's going well? Tell me about life…."

2. Listen for understanding (as opposed to listening briefly and then offering information right away).

3. Elicit their story: It's important to elicit not only what's going on in adolescents' lives, but also their values and beliefs, even their future goals for themselves.

4. Express empathy. When they discuss the difficulties of behavioral change, it's critical that we acknowledge these.

   "Given that smoking is your only way of relieving stress, I can see why it would be hard to give it up."

5. Develop discrepancy. Reflect back the teen's own ambivalence about change.

   "So on the one hand…but on the other hand…."

6. Resist the "righting reflex." Don't argue why the teen should do something. Remember, this naturally creates resistance, making adolescents feel compelled to say why they can't. Remember, it's *their* job to present argument for change, not ours!

7. Reflect back resistance. If a teen doesn't seem to want to engage in the conversation at all, name what you see.

   "It looks like you really don't want to be here today."
   "It sounds like it's impossible for you to check your sugars four times a day."

8. Allow silence. Elaborate on their resistance.

   "What makes it so hard?"
   "What would help?"

9. Support self-efficacy. This is done by pointing out successes.

   "Wow. You quit smoking for 2 whole weeks…that's tremendous."

10. Explore self-efficacy:

    "So how did you resist the urge to light up a cigarette when it happened? What did you do instead?"

    Have the youth brainstorm with you about overcoming triggers in the future.

11. Explore triggers for relapse (either past or future).

    "When did you have that first cigarette again? What pushed you over? If that were to occur again, what do you think you could you do in the future to resist the urge?"

12. Support the teen in defining a treatment plan and commitment to change.

    "What do you think about trying again? When do you want to try? When would you like to check in again?"

■ Evoking "Change Talk" (Specific Tools)

There are several interviewing "tools" that have been developed over the years to assist in getting youth to identify their desire and ability to change the target behavior. A few of these are explored as follows, using some of the principles described above:

Elaborating

Understand the teen's world view. As mentioned above, it's very helpful to start with a general psychosocial screen before asking specifics about the issue at hand. Then explore the issue using open-ended questions.

> *"Tell me about your diabetes. How does it affect the rest of your life?"*
>
> *"Tell me about your (behavior). When did it start?"*
>
> *"How do you feel about it?"*
>
> *"What do you get out of (problem behavior)?"*
>
> *"How do you think it causes difficulties for you?"*

Express Empathy

> *"I can see why it must be hard for you…."*

Develop discrepancy between the polarized urges (summarize ambivalence by reflecting back pros and cons).

> *"So on one hand…and on the other…."*
>
> *"Part of you wants…and the other part…."*

Using the "Importance" Ruler

There are 3 parts to using the importance ruler (see Figure 11-1). The first part is as follows:

> *"On a scale of 1 to 10, 10 being 'absolutely yes' and 1 being 'not at all,' how motivated are you to _____(check your sugars at school)?"*

Ten is always the direction in which you want the change to go.

The second part is to then explore whatever number the teen gives you. If she picked "5," elect 1 or 2 numbers *below* and ask: *"Why a 5? Why not a 3?"* By choosing a number below the one she picked, you are eliciting "change talk" (getting her to describe what her reasons are for changing).

The third part is to then take a number or 2 above what she gave you and ask, *"What would it take to move you to a 6 (not actually changing the behavior, but a little more comfortable with the idea)?"* Be sure to elicit something the teen has control over. Whatever the adolescent tells you may become the treatment plan. Remember, it is critical to make sure the plan is something that can actually be accomplished. Work with the youth to explore potential barriers to the plan and appropriate solutions:

> *"What do you think might get in the way?"*
>
> *"What could you do to ensure that it doesn't?"*

Have the teen set an appropriate timeline for implementing the plan.

Sometimes the issue is not importance or motivation, but confidence that she will be able to make the change. An example of this might be weight loss. Use the same strategy, only as a "confidence" ruler:

> *"On a scale from 1 to 10, how confident are you that you could…?"*

If you don't distinguish between these 2 (importance vs confidence), you may inadvertently explore the wrong idea with the youth, who will consequently disengage from the conversation. One strategy is to explore both.

FIGURE 11.1
READINESS, IMPORTANCE, AND
CONFIDENCE RULERS

Readiness, Importance and Confidence Rulers

READINESS: On a scale from 1 to 10, with 10 being very ready, how ready are you to make a change?

1	2	3	4	5	6	7	8	9	10
Not at all				Somewhat					Very

IMPORTANCE: On a scale of 1 to 10, with 10 being very important, how important is it for you to change?

1	2	3	4	5	6	7	8	9	10
Not at all				Somewhat					Very

CONFIDENCE: On a scale of 1 to 10, with 10 begin very interested, how interested are you in changing?

1	2	3	4	5	6	7	8	9	10
Not at all				Somewhat					Very

Adapted with permission from Gold MA, Kokotailo PK. Motivational interviewing strategies to facilitate adolescent behavior change. *Adolescent Health Update.* 2007;20(1)

Similar rulers can be found at the listed reference above.

Querying Extremes

Always start by exploring the youth's feelings about the *current* behavior.

If the behavior is undesired or a "problem", start by asking, *"What's the best thing about it?"* Then ask *"What's the worst thing about it?"* That way, the youth feels understood as to why the behavior change is difficult at the beginning of the conversation before exploring what might be advantages and benefits to changing their behavior.

If the behavior is desired or the "solution," start by asking, *"What's the worst thing about it?"*

Hopefully, that will help the youth also be able to discuss what is good about the desired behavior.

Exploring Goals and Values

There are 2 parts to this tool: exploring goals and values, and exploring how the current behavior fits with those goals and values:

1. *"What things are most important to you in your life right now?"* (You may want to do a general psychosocial screen, such as SSHADESS.) Then reflect back what is said: *"It sounds like being able to do what your friends do is important to you."*

2. The second part is to then explore how the current behavior is affecting this value or goal.

   "How do you think (diagnosis/current behavior) fits with these goals/values?"

   "How can you minimize (the problem) so it doesn't get in the way of living your life the way you want/fully?"

Your tone of voice must be gentle and exploratory, and not critical, in order for this approach to be successful. This technique alone has been most highly correlated with behavioral change; understandable since the youth begins to realize that his current behavior is not in alignment with his *own* values and beliefs.

Elicit-Provide-Elicit

Sometimes we still need to give information and advice. How do we do this without creating resistance? A very powerful way of maintaining openness while receiving information is to simply *ask* for permission before giving advice. This supports the young person's sense of autonomy.

"Of course, while I can only suggest, you're ultimately the one to decide...."

It is also helpful to first elicit what the youth knows about the topic to be discussed, and offer praise for whatever is known **(Elicit).**

"What do you know about (health condition/problem behavior, etc)"? "It sounds like you know quite a bit about...."

Next, you ask for permission to share further information **(Provide).**

"There is some other information that might be helpful to you...may I share that with you?"

Finally, you explore how the information you provided was received **(Elicit).**

"What are your thoughts about that? How might you use that information? Is there anything that might be relevant for you?"

When given permission to offer suggestions, it's often helpful to offer several strategies. If you offer only one suggestion, it looks like the "right" answer, and it will create resistance. It might inadvertently drive the young person to offer reasons why it won't work.

"Here are some ideas...which one do you think might work best for you? Tell me more."

In the case of weight loss,

"Which would you like to work on first: healthy food choices, moving your body more, or reducing your stress levels?"

"How would you like to achieve this?"

"When would you like to start?"

"When would you like to come back and see me?"

If you offer solutions one at a time, it too creates resistance, and the young person may be more likely to offer reasons why each one won't work.

■ FRAMES

A mnemonic that may be particularly useful for those new to motivational interviewing is FRAMES. This brief adaptation of MI may be useful for helping a young person move into action and make a needed change, especially when time is limited.

1. **Feedback:** Offer personalized information about a behavior. For example, *"You told me that you are drinking alcohol almost every weekend at parties and that you are worried that it is too much for someone your age. You are right that drinking alcohol is not the safest thing for a teenager to be doing because it impairs your thinking and can lead to some unsafe decisions."*

2. **Responsibility:** Emphasize the young person's autonomy. *"Of course, in the end, it's up to you to decide if you are going to stop drinking alcohol."*

3. **Advice:** Ask permission and then offer clear recommendations based on your own experience. For example, after gaining permission to share ideas, you can say, *"In my experience it is most helpful for people your age to stop drinking altogether because even small amounts of alcohol can be problematic. Sometimes people find it helpful to not be around alcohol for a while, say a few weeks, until they feel confident in their ability not to drink. What do you think about that? Is that something you might be interested in trying?"*

4. **Menu:** Elicit options for change and help the young person develop a list of potential methods for change. By eliciting suggestions from her and by identifying several options you support the young person's autonomy to make a decision about the strategy she feels is best for her. For example, *"So we talked about ways to help you stop drinking alcohol. You can ask your friends not to drink around you. You can stay at home and watch movies with your sister when you know there will be drinking at a party. Or you can bring a soda with you to drink instead."*

5. **Empathy:** Remain nonjudgmental and show your support for the young person regardless of how ready she is to change. For example, *"It must be really hard to choose not to drink when all of your friends are doing it."*

6. **Self-efficacy:** Support the young person's strengths and reinforce her ability to make changes. For example, you might ask, *"Let's talk about times in the past where you had to do something that was hard, like learning to play a new sport or musical instrument. Maybe together we can figure out how you were successful and how you can use those same skills to help you reach your goal of not drinking so much."*

■ OARES

Another mnemonic that incorporates key MI communication components is OARES: **o**pen-ended questions, **a**ffirmation, **r**eflective listening, **e**licit change talk, and **s**ummarizing. This technique may be especially useful in initial encounters, ▶11.3 when developing rapport and attempting to demonstrate support of the young person's autonomy and self-efficacy.

■ Motivational Interviewing and Adolescent Development

Using MI with adolescents is particularly important, since it is *critical* to engage them in decision-making and treatment planning for developmental reasons.

1. Adolescents begin to shift from the concrete thinking of childhood to the more abstract, sophisticated thinking of adulthood, causing them to want to be seen as part of the solution, not just the problem.

2. Their sense of self (identity formation) becomes front and center, as do the development of their personal values and beliefs.

3. A desire for autonomy/individuation and resistance to being told what to do emerges during adolescence. (It doesn't necessarily resolve later in life, explaining why adults, too, are often resistant to advice about changing behaviors!)

■ Remember

Stress physiology and subsequent distorted cognition are often driving the "problem behavior" (see Chapter 6).

When stress is managed in a healthier, prosocial way, the need to use problem behavior as a coping strategy diminishes (see Chapter 8).

●● Group Learning and Discussion ●●

In the following scenarios, how might each of the following techniques be used to explore behavior change in young people: Elaborating? Confidence ruler? Querying extremes? Elicit-provide-elicit? FRAMES? Break into pairs and work through these scenarios.

1. A 16-year-old comes to see you for a sports physical examination. During the conversation, when asked if she smokes cigarettes, she states, *"Only at parties."* How could you explore her smoking behavior further using open-ended questions?

2. A 17-year-old shares that he wishes he could lose weight, but doesn't think he can. How might you explore this issue further using open-ended questions?

3. A 15-year-old is struggling with managing her time more efficiently so that she can get to sleep early enough so that she's not so tired "all the time." How might an adult in her life help her understand what the barriers are to her getting to bed on time?

■ Reference

1. Prochaska JO, DiClemente CC. Stages of change in the modification of problem behaviors. *Prog Behav Modif.* 1992;28:183

■ Suggested Reading

Levy S, Knight JR. Office-based management of adolescent substance use and abuse. In: Neinstein LS, Gordon CM, Katzman DK, Rosen DS, Woods ER, eds. *Adolescent Health Care: A Practical Guide.* 5th ed. Philadelphia, PA: Lippincott, Williams and Wilkins; 2007

Miller WR, Rollnick S. *Motivational Interviewing: Preparing People to Change.* New York, NY: Guilford Press; 2002

Miller WR, Rollnick S. *What's New Since MI-2? Stockholm, Sweden, June 2010.* http://www.motivationalinterview.org/Documents/Miller-and-Rollnick-june6-pre-conference-workshop.pdf. Accessed June 25, 2013

Miller WR, Sanches VC. Motivating young adults for treatment and lifestyle change. In: Howard GS, Nathan PE, eds. *Alcohol Use and Misuse by Young Adults.* Notre Dame, IN: University of Notre Dame Press; 1994

Naar-King S, Suarez M. *Motivational Interviewing With Adolescents and Young Adults.* New York, NY: The Guilford Press; 2011

Rollnick S, Miller WR, Butler CC. *Motivational Interviewing in Health Care: Helping Patients Change Behavior.* New York, NY: The Guilford Press; 2008

■ Related Video Content

11.0 Motivational Interviewing With Adolescents. Singh.

11.1 Motivational Interviewing With a Young Woman With an Eating Disorder. Kreipe.

11.2 Motivational Interviewing: Making Sure to Uncover the Teen's Perspective. Singh.

11.3 Motivational Interviewing: OARS. Kinsman.

11.4 Using Motivational Interviewing to Help Substance-Using Youth Consider Change. Pletcher.

11.5 Case: Motivational Interviewing in Substance-Using Youth. Singh.

■ Related Web Site

Motivational Interviewing
www.motivationalinterview.org

Strategies to Help Adolescents Own Their Solutions

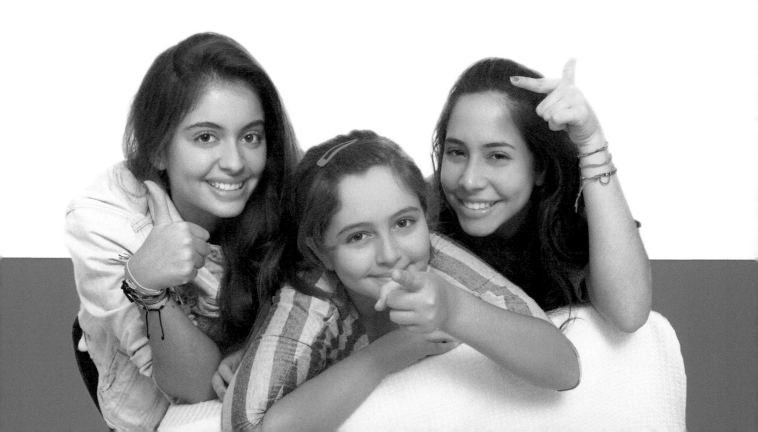

CHAPTER 12

Helping Adolescents Own Their Solutions

Kenneth R. Ginsburg, MD, MS Ed, FAAP, FSAHM

 Related Video Content

12.0 Facilitating Adolescents to Own Their Solution: Replacing the Lecture With Youth-Driven Strategies

■ Why This Matters

Young people have repeated experiences being told what to do. In their quest for independence, they become resentful toward adults informing them of their unwise decision-making skills and can be reflexively resistant, if not rebellious, against the guidance. To steer youth away from risk behaviors and toward healthier behaviors, we have to be able to deliver information in an engaging and informative, rather than alienating, manner.

The ultimate goal of any information exchange is for teens to reach their own healthy conclusions. When teens "own" the solution, they have nothing to be resistant against. In contrast, when we impose our solutions on them, we undermine their sense of competence by communicating, *"I don't think you can handle this."*

There is another reason young people resist adult guidance: They don't understand it and naturally reject advice that makes them feel stupid or incapable. This is because most adult guidance is offered through a lecture. The intentions are good, but lectures backfire because youth cannot absorb their content.

> **Young people reject adult guidance they don't understand and rebel against advice that makes them feel incapable. When they own their solutions, they want to follow through on *their* plans.**

■ Helping Youth Arrive at Their Own Conclusions

To appreciate why youth may not get reasonable cause-and-effect lectures, we must consider how they think. Children and early adolescents think concretely; as they grow, they become more capable of understanding abstract concepts.[1,2] Then, they become capable of imagining the future and recognize how choices they make in the present lead to different future outcomes. Most teens in mid- to late adolescence are abstract thinkers, but some teens of below average intelligence will never get there. It is also critical to understand that *all* people think concretely during times of extreme stress,[3] and, in our professional settings, we are often dealing with people under acute stress.

Now let's break down a typical lecture.

- *"What you are doing now, let's call it behavior A, will very likely lead to consequence B. And then consequence B will go on to consequence C, which almost always ends up with D happening! At this point, you'll likely lose control, making you much more vulnerable to consequence E.* [If it is a parent doing the lecturing, add here, *"Look at me when I'm talking to you, I'm not talking for my own good!!"*] *Then, depending on several factors likely out of your control, consequence F, G, or H will happen. I may even happen. Do you know what happens if I happens? You might die!"*

We lecture to spare youth the fate of learning through painful life lessons. But, the typical lecture has an algebraic pattern—variables affect outcomes in mysterious ways. Algebra isn't taught to pre- or early adolescents because their brains aren't ready for abstract thinking. And a person in crisis wants to be running; they really shouldn't be contemplating algebra. When we lecture young people, they become frustrated because they're not yet capable of following our thoughts. They hear our concern but not the content of our message.

Our challenge is to deliver information so that youth can figure things out themselves. If they do, the lesson is more likely to be long lasting and to reinforce their motivation.

Early adolescents (and people in crisis) can grasp information if it is delivered in a more concrete, mathematical cadence—like 2 plus 2 equals 4. They can better follow our reasoning if instead of a string of abstract possibilities (A to B to C to D), the lesson is broken down into separate steps. *"I appreciate your desire to do A, but I am worried A might lead to B. Do you have any experience with something like that? Tell me about that experience. What might you do to make sure that doesn't happen to you? Do you see how B might lead to C? Have you ever seen that happen? What are your plans to avoid that happening here?"* We congratulate them and reinforce their existing plans to be safe and healthy. We pause at each step as they figure things out that they had not previously considered. They are the experts in their own lives. We are only the facilitators.

This approach increases competence because we're asking youth to consider possible consequences step by step with their own thoughts, based on their own experiences, rather than through scenarios we dictate. They may better learn the lessons because they have figured them out.

Here are some specific techniques you might use to guide adolescents to recognize consequences and generate their own solutions.

■ Choreographed Conversations

This is the most casual way to teach problem-solving and build competence. Like choreography, it should appear spontaneous but be thoughtfully planned. This technique was described above.

Role-playing

Role-playing allows youth to arrive at their own conclusions. This strategy also allows them to explore hypothetical situations and grasp how their decisions or actions determine outcomes. It is important to set up role-playing casually. If you suggest, *"Let's role-play, "* they may quickly seek an exit. Instead, be subtle and work *"what if..."* and *"what'll happen when..."* scenarios into your conversations. Keep the tone light and avoid confrontational dialogue. Don't jump in with answers. Role-playing is an ideal way to teach social skills.

- For example, you have just done a SSHADESS screen and learned that older kids have approached Yael, a 12-year-old, to try marijuana. Rather than telling her, *"Lets role-play what you should say,"* you might start with, *"Well, older kids do sometimes try to influence younger kids, but you can be well prepared."* An eighth grader might come up to you and say, *"All the cooler kids are already smoking weed, you seem pretty cool for a sixth grader, have you tried it yet?"* What might you say?

Decision Trees

A decision tree allows you to transform the choreographed conversation onto paper (Figure 12.1). It makes the lesson even more concrete and allows the young person to leave the office with lesson in hand.

The decision tree can be used with a variety of scenarios including, *"What will happen to you if you become pregnant?" "Where does using drugs lead you?" "Where does putting in a really good effort in school now lead you to?"* and *"I know you're angry, but what will happen if you fight?"*

The ladder diagram described in Chapter 13 is one form of a decision tree.

Case Example 12.2

A 14-year-old female presented with blood on her eye to a school-based clinic. She had been in a fight the day before with a classmate who insulted her mother.

When asked what was going to happen next, she responded, *"I'm going to kill her, that's why I brought this knife* [which she had in her pocket] *to school."*

- A lecture may have backfired and possibly created a hostile exchange between the doctor and this knife-wielding patient. Instead, it was calmly requested that the girl keep the knife in her pocket and role-play the possible scenarios with a marker substituting as a knife. At each point the doctor wrote down her response into an evolving decision tree. He asked short questions and allowed her to respond thoughtfully and at her own pace.
- At first, she was guided to walk through various scenarios to grasp the fact that the knife could be turned on her with serious consequences.

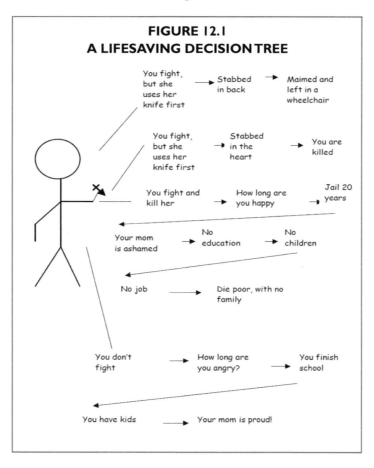

FIGURE 12.1
A LIFESAVING DECISION TREE

- Then she was allowed to imagine that she had successfully killed the intended victim. When asked how that would make her feel. She responded, *"Good!"* When asked how long she would feel good she responded, *"All day!"* She was then guided to consider how her actions would affect her mother, since she was getting into this fight to protect her mother's honor. The next steps in this path are illustrated on the accompanying decision tree.
- Finally, the girl was asked to consider how she would feel if she did not get into the fight. She responded, *"Angry!"* When asked how long she would feel angry she responded, *"All day!"* When she realized that this path led to children, an education, and making her mother proud, the choice became clear.

This girl needed a technique that would allow her to contemplate future consequences in the safety of an office, rather than the realities of the street. It convinced her to engage in a process of conflict resolution. She owned the solution and wanted to follow through on her plans.

■ Final Thought

You don't have to learn anything new to begin implementing these strategies and help adolescents own their own solutions. You already have the wisdom that connects their actions to long term consequences. The only thing you may need to do is change the cadence with which you deliver the information from an abstract lecture to a concrete step-by-step technique.

•• Group Learning and Discussion ••

You do not have to learn new content to improve on the wisdom and advice you have been sharing. Your challenge is to change the delivery style so that young people figure things out by themselves (aided with your facilitation) so that they own the solutions.

In a group setting, recall some cases where you needed to guide a young person toward safer behaviors. Then break into pairs and practice using choreographed conversations, role-playing, or decision trees to facilitate youth thinking. If you prefer, you can use the following cases.

1. Emily is a 16-year-old who wants to get pregnant. She states, *"I am so ready to love my baby. My boyfriend will make the best father. My mother had me at 17 and she may have struggled, but she is a great mom and has given me everything I ever needed."*

2. LaVon was in a fight yesterday. He got jumped by 3 guys. He knows that they will get him again until he proves he's not a punk. He is thinking about getting even. But, he's not going to be unprepared. He knows where to get a switchblade.

3. Nathan is 15 and hates school. He can't wait until he turns 16 so he can drop out. He'll just get a job. No one at school cares about teaching. They don't teach what he needs anyway. He wants to be a car mechanic and he's great with his hands and can take things apart and put them back together easily. (FYI, you live in a mid-sized city with 6 high schools, including one that focuses on vocational technical education.)

References

1. Piaget J. *The Child's Conception of the World.* London, United Kingdom: Routledge and Kegan Paul; 1951
2. Pandit A, Archana, Raman V, Ashok MV. Developmental pediatrics. In: Bhat SR, ed. *Achar's Textbook of Pediatrics.* 4th ed. Andhra Pradesh, India: University Press; 2009
3. Horowitz MJ. Cognitive response to stress and experimental demand. *J Abnorm Psychol.* 1971;78(1):86–92

Related Video Content

12.0 Facilitating Adolescents to Own Their Solution: Replacing the Lecture With Youth-Driven Strategies. Ginsburg.

12.1 Teens Told What They "Should" Do Will Lose the Ability to Learn What They Can Do. Rich.

12.2 Helping a Young Person Own Her Solution: A Case of Using a Decision Tree to Prevent Violent Retaliation. Ginsburg.

12.3 Guiding Parents and Teens to Understand the Shifting Balance Between Parental Control and Teen Decision-Making. Sugerman.

Related Handout/Supplementary Material

Stop Lecturing: Guiding Adolescents to Make Their Own Wise Decisions

CHAPTER 13

Gaining a Sense of Control—One Step at a Time

Kenneth R. Ginsburg, MD, MS Ed, FAAP, FSAHM

 Related Video Content

13.0 Gaining a Sense of Control: One Step at a Time

■ Why This Matters

Sometimes a decision to move toward a new positive behavior seems so overwhelming or a goal so elusive that young people don't even consider trying.[1] They feel frightened and frustrated by their powerlessness. They convince themselves that they have no choices. They believe they're controlled by outside forces that determine their destiny—they have an external locus of control.[2-4]

When young people feel incapable of changing, we can offer a relatively brief intervention that may help them get past the mental block that serves as a major barrier to contemplating change. This technique is designed to help a young person revisualize a problem into manageable steps and then, perhaps, even to experience a moment of competence in their decision to consider action. Even the brief experience with success may give a youth enough of a sense of control to consider further steps.

> **We can help a young person revisualize a problem into manageable steps and then, perhaps, even to experience a moment of competence in their decision to consider action. Even a brief experience with success may give a youth enough of a sense of control to consider further steps.**

■ It Is Stressful to Feel Powerless

A sense of powerlessness increases one's stress. Some of the most effective stress reduction strategies are those that are problem-focused, because they help an individual to address, manage, and hopefully diminish a problem.

In the 10-point stress reduction plan offered in Chapter 8, point 1 is to identify and then address the problem. A key to using this strategy is to clarify the problem and then divide it into smaller pieces, committing to work on only one piece at a time. This decreases the sense of being overwhelmed and increases efficacy. **▶8.2**

Metaphorically, this is about helping teens revisualize problems from being mountains too high to be scaled into hills situated on top of each other. As they stand atop each hill, the summit appears more attainable.

The ladder technique is one strategy that can be used to help teens approach larger crises or emotional issues by breaking them into manageable steps. Consequently, it may also increase one's internal locus of control.

■ The Ladder Technique

The ladder technique can be used with adolescents who never thought they could succeed in school or never considered that they could become healthier by losing weight or exercising. It's been used with young people burdened with drug addiction or trapped in gangs. All of these groups have in common the sense of being so "stuck" that they don't believe they have control over their lives. It is about focusing on one step at a time so that a teen can revisualize a problem from being too large to manage into one that can be tackled.

Many teens can only consider one step at a time and may need to return another day to consider next steps. In fact, a teen who is steeped in a sense of powerlessness may not even be able to come up with the very first step. Invite him to come back anyway. Even if he returns still unable to imagine the first step, you can reinforce that just the act of returning *is* a step. The acknowledgment that he is choosing to move forward can be powerful in itself and may "unblock" his creative juices and, therefore, facilitate further action.

- **Step 1:** When you sense the adolescent is too stuck to even consider the possibility of change, explain that all people get overwhelmed and have moments when they can't imagine taking any steps that would actually make a difference.
- **Step 2:** Help the teen to think about where he is presently. Draw that present state as the base of a diagram; it can even just be called "Today."
- **Step 3:** Tell the teen that you certainly don't have the answers but hope he can find them himself.
- **Step 4:** Tell him that after listening to him you do know there are a couple of different possible futures for him. Write them at the top ends of 2 separate ladders leading to 2 distant but real destinations. One is the positive, hopeful future and the other is the future he hopes to avoid. This is not a threat; in fact, the positive future should reflect precisely his stated goals. Use all of the strengths you have elicited about him to make him know that you sincerely believe in his potential to reach that goal.
- **Step 5:** Repeat that, while you don't have the solutions, you do know that each ladder has several rungs along the way, and that everyone climbs a ladder one step at a time before they reach the top. Sometimes people don't even look to the top, they just know that if they hold on and find their balance they can take one step at a time.
- **Step 6:** Ask the teen to suggest what steps will lead to the less desirable end. Because he's feeling overwhelmed and helpless, he may know precisely which steps lead to the negative outcome. Unfortunately, he may feel he has mastered those decisions and actions.
- **Step 7:** Challenge him to visualize even the first step on the positive path and ideally help him achieve mastery over that first step.
- **Step 8:** As he attempts to write the steps toward the positive endpoint, remind him how much easier it is to divide difficult tasks into many small steps. Guide him to keep his eye on the future dream to stay motivated, but focus on only one step at a time to avoid feeling overwhelmed.

Cases

Case 1

Felipe is an 11-year-old morbidly obese boy who is unable to participate in sports because he is unable to keep up with his peers. His parents are obese but nag him to lose weight, and his peers tease him. He desperately wants to lose weight, but can only admit that while looking at the floor. Until his conversation in the office, he has never even talked about how much he wanted to lose weight. Instead, he became hostile when people brought up weight: *"I don't care. Why should you?"* He confides that he's failed every time he's tried to lose weight in the past. He doesn't even want to try again; he knows he will fail.

- The clinician sketched out the 2 ladders and asked what steps Felipe had to take to continue gaining weight. He knew exactly the unhealthy habits that were leading to his obesity. These habits were written on different rungs.
- Then he was asked to name only one step he could take toward a healthier path. He was assured that once he just mastered one step, each successive step would seem easier. Felipe struggled at first to come up with a single step, explaining with each option what would get in the way, why he would fail. He eventually decided that he could stop drinking sugary drinks and replace them with water and diet drinks.
- When he returned to the clinician's office a month later, he had lost 3 pounds! More importantly, he realized that food did not control him; rather, he controlled what he ate. He realized he could follow through on a decision. This experience of self-control gave him the confidence to contemplate his next step and then to put it into action. He began taking walks.

Case 2

Tori is a 14-year-old girl trapped in a gang run by her 16-year-old female cousin. She is a bright, engaging girl who was too overwhelmed to escape her dangerous circumstances. She wants to become an architect when she gets older because she hopes to build buildings in her community to keep neighborhood children off the streets. Every effort at counseling from the clinician was met with resistance. She repeatedly stated, *"You don't know what you are talking about. That's family!"* She didn't say this with hostility, just with a pervasive sense of hopelessness.

- The ladder diagram (Figure 13.1) allowed Tori to visualize her different futures. She knew precisely which steps would continue to lead her toward trouble and maybe even death.
- The ladder technique allowed the abstract concept of *"you need to turn your life around"* to be divided into much smaller concrete steps. Nevertheless, on her first visit she was unable to even name the first steps on the positive ladder. She did agree, however, to return for a check-in the next week.
- She returned and voiced her embarrassment that she couldn't even think of one right step. She told the clinician, *"I failed you. I took this out every night and all I could see was me headed down the wrong path."* She was told that just returning was a very positive step. This simple realization allowed her to realize that she did have some control over her decisions. This instantly belied her belief that she was powerless, trapped by her fellow gang members.

The same girl who spent the week unable to come up with any possibilities immediately began generating ideas. She needed her mother to help her navigate her away from the gang. Her cousin loved and respected her mother (that was family too!) and would allow Tori to have that relationship. Tori's mother was engaged in the plan using a strength-based approach. In a *"just blame me"* conspiracy, Tori would call her

▶ 13.1

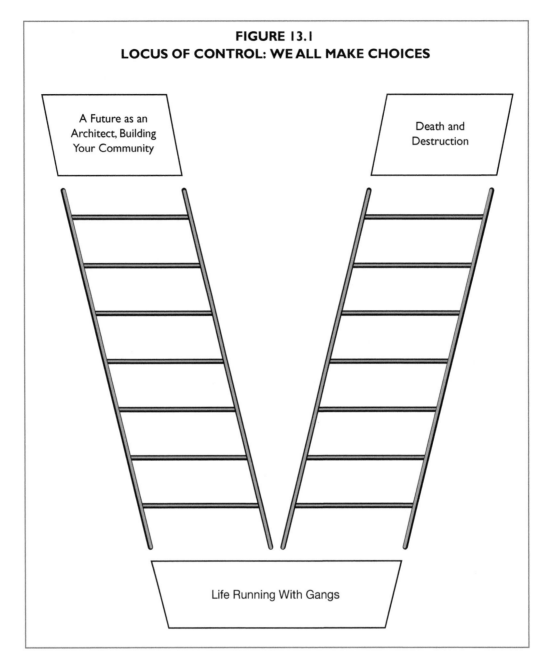

FIGURE 13.1
LOCUS OF CONTROL: WE ALL MAKE CHOICES

A Future as an Architect, Building Your Community

Death and Destruction

Life Running With Gangs

mother when she was in a potentially dangerous gang scenario. Her mother would recognize the "code word" and then demand that she come home (see Chapter 3, page 23). Ultimately, they moved a couple of miles away, enough of a distance to be out of gang territory. Tori was able to leave the gang and later attended college.

■ Final Thoughts

This brief office-based intervention facilitates adolescents to overcome their sense of powerlessness, their lack of control, and their belief that only fate determines their futures. A pattern of repeated failures that stifles contemplation toward change can sometimes be broken when even a small success is experienced.

•• Group Learning and Discussion ••

Discuss cases in which teens felt powerless and strategies you have used to help them gain a sense of control. Either use those cases or choose from those below to practice creating a ladder diagram so youth can learn to achieve success a step at a time. Feel free to assume that your conversation occurs over several weeks.

Case 1: Aamina is a 14-year-old young woman who has tried "everything" to lose weight, but has never succeeded. She has even gained weight after every effort. She thinks that is because she eats more when she is frustrated.

Case 2: Grayson has never done well in school. When he was 16 years old, he dropped out as soon as it became legal to do so. He "lived the life" for a while, but wants to be able to have a family one day and have kids who would be proud of him. He would love to be a mechanic. He can't imagine going through the applications or even getting started. He had one teacher who said that he had attention-deficit/hyperactivity disorder, but he never told his mom.

Case 3: Dalia was always a very good student. She got straight As, volunteered in a neighborhood animal shelter, and had dreamed of going to a top college. Her parents are immigrants and want her to get her education, but were never able to receive theirs. They push her at home, but have never gone into a school meeting. Dalia is in 11th grade and her friends are applying to colleges. She has a meeting with her school counselor in 6 weeks. She says it is "all stupid" and tells you that her cousins are doing fine in the family business. Her grades are dropping.

■ References

1. Schwarzer R, Fuchs R. Changing risk behaviors and adopting health behaviors: the role of self-efficacy beliefs. In: Bandura A, ed. *Self-Efficacy in Changing Societies*. Cambridge, United Kingdom: Cambridge University Press; 1997
2. Rotter, JB. *Social Learning and Clinical Psychology*. Upper Saddle River, NJ: Prentice-Hall; 1954
3. Rotter JB. Generalized expectancies of internal versus external control of reinforcements. *Psychol Monogr*. 1966;80:609
4. Lefcourt HM. Internal versus external control of reinforcement: a review. *Psychol Bull*. 1966;65(4):206–220

■ Related Video Content

13.0 Gaining a Sense of Control: One Step at a Time. Ginsburg.

13.1 Delivering Upsetting News to Parents: Recognizing Their Strengths First. Ginsburg.

8.2 Stress Management and Coping/Section 1/Tackling the Problem. Ginsburg.

Delivering Bad News in a Way That May Buffer Inevitable Stress

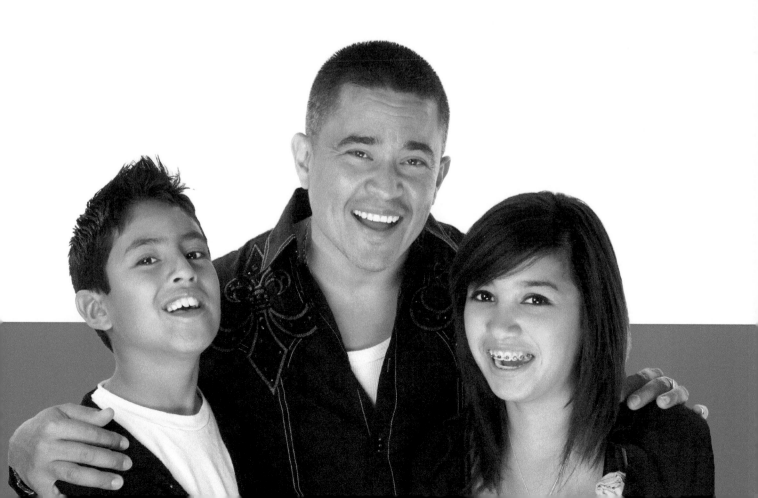

CHAPTER 14

Delivering Bad News to Adolescents

Daniel H. Reirden, MD, FAAP, AAHIVMS
Kenneth R. Ginsburg, MD, MS Ed, FAAP, FSAHM

 Related Video Content

14.0 Among the Hardest Things We Do—Delivering Bad News

■ Why This Matters

As we care for adolescents, we often have to share news that they would rather not hear. There is no way to make these disclosures pleasant, but we can make a difference in the adolescents' experience. How they experience receiving the news may make a large difference in the next steps they take (or don't take) to address the issue. If they experience shame or stigma, they may reject further services. If they are left feeling without hope, they may catastrophize the situation and move into denial, or, worse, entertain self-harm. On the other hand, if they feel cared for and about, they may engage in a relationship that will enable you to guide them toward the best outcome.

> **As important as it is to make yourself available for follow-up, it is even more vital not to overpromise. Many youth have experience with adults who have been inconsistent and unavailable; you do not want to be added to that list. Be clear and honest about your service and limitations.**

■ Tips for Breaking Bad News

The following tips are not meant to feel formulaic or to constitute a recipe. Rather they are general thoughts for your consideration.

1. *Consider your own reaction prior to working with the youth or family.* It is normal, even desirable, to be genuinely saddened by news that you know will alter a teen's life direction. In some cases, you might be particularly shocked if, for some reason, you related closely to the youth. In other cases, you may need to work through a sense of guilt or responsibility for not having prevented the problem. All of these feelings are reasonable and normal, but have to be resolved before you interact with the youth because he or she will read your affect and that will alter the experience. The youth should not feel as though he or she needs to care for you.

2. *Decide if you are the best person to break the news.* It is okay to determine that a colleague has a better relationship with the youth or more expertise in a specific area. However, this can only be done in a setting where the colleague would naturally be exposed to the information; confidentiality remains a paramount issue. Further, a teen may experience another caregiver delivering the news as being passed off or may conclude that you consider the issue stigmatizing. Depending on your assessment of

these considerations, you can have the colleague with the longstanding relationship be available for partnering with you if the youth requests it.

3. *Practice what you will say.* This is especially important if this is a difficult topic for you or the news raises strong feelings in you. Stumbling with the news will raise the youth's anxiety about the gravity of the situation.

4. *Consider who should be present.* Is there someone that the youth would like to be there for emotional support? Are there key members of the care team who should be present?

5. *Assess the physical space.* Select a space that is as quiet and private as possible. Arrange to have adequate time to spend with the teen, and make every attempt to limit interruptions during this period. Making sure that you're prepared with items, such as tissues, conveys a message that you have thought about the youth's emotional needs beforehand. Sit down when you deliver the news. Do not block an exit from the room, as people who receive concerning news often have a need to flee. Although people almost universally control this instinctual impulse, if an exit is blocked, it can reinforce the sense of being trapped.

6. *Be prepared for escalations.* If the news is likely to create an angry response, (eg, a murder of a friend) or if the youth has a history of volatile reactions, have a safety plan in place. A colleague, or security if appropriate, should know the timing and location of the disclosure and you should be certain that the exit is not blocked for you. Be prepared to de-escalate the situation, with the initial step always being listening without judgment (see Chapter 15).

7. *Be conscious of your body language.* Remember that about 80% of what we communicate is conveyed nonverbally. All of your preparation and practice in finding the right words to say can be undermined by your body language. Take deep breaths or practice mindfulness techniques to stabilize your emotions before entering the room. Then be conscious of your body language as youth, particularly marginalized adolescents, are acutely sensitive to body language that conveys fear or judgment. Your body language, which may actually be associated with your own discomfort or sadness, may be misinterpreted as being judgmental. It is important, therefore, to maintain an open, calm body posture. ▶9.3

8. *Be direct.* Beating around the bush or engaging in prolonged small talk will increase anxiety and generate confusion. Be calm and gentle, but come to the point quickly. Avoid retreating to the professional comfort zone of offering technical details rather than attending to the youth's emotional needs. If you are providing bad news related to a medical condition, it can be extremely helpful to assess what the teen's understanding of the situation is prior to disclosing the news. You might say something like, *"I want to get a sense of what you remember about why we got this particular medical test."* You may have a sentence that emotionally prepares the youth to listen carefully. *"I have some bad/upsetting news to share with you today."* Then, share the news gently and directly. *"I am sorry to have to tell you that there was a terrible crash today, and _____ was killed." "I am sorry to tell you that your HIV test was positive, meaning that you are infected with HIV." "I am so sorry to tell you that there was a gang shooting earlier in the day, and _____ was killed."* If the bad news is related to a medical diagnosis, asking about how much detail/information the youth wants in that moment can be helpful. In the case of test results, have written proof available, as youth often request to see it.

9. *Allow time for initial reaction.* The emotions may be shock, anger, or denial. None of them are wrong. This is the time to listen. If the teen doesn't respond immediately, the importance of allowing a period of silence to occur cannot be overemphasized. During this time, maintain an open, calm body posture and remain connected to the teen by not looking away. After a suitable period of silence, an open-ended question, such

as, *"Tell me how you're feeling right now,"* or *"What's going on in your head?"* can help facilitate further conversation.

Never minimize an emotion by saying, *"I understand,"* or *"It isn't that bad."* Just listen. When you do say something, make the connection between the reaction and the news. This will validate the emotions and make it clear that you see their reaction as connected to the news and are not judging it. *"This is clearly shocking news, and I see how angry you are."* Do not be shocked, yourself, if the news does not seem to shake the youth. Sometimes in the context of a hectic life, a youth may not view a situation in the same catastrophic manner that you would in the same situation. One of the reasons it is so important that you control your own verbal and nonverbal messages is that otherwise you can convey a sense of catastrophe that a youth may not have experienced.

10. *Appropriate touching.* Touch needs to be used judiciously, leaving absolutely no room for misinterpretation, because we need to assume the possibility that the young person has been exposed to inappropriate touch. If an adolescent is weeping silently, a hand on the youth's shoulder or hand can be an appropriate way to reinforce that you are fully present. In the case of a young person receiving news of a condition that is stigmatizing (eg, HIV or other sexually transmitted infection), touch can contribute to healing because it conveys that you do not see the young person as somehow tainted.

11. *Convey messages of hope whenever possible.* Sometimes the most hopeful message you can convey is that *"You'll get through this."* But even that message may not feel helpful in the case of the news of a death. On the other hand, in the case of news about illness like HIV or cancer, it is important to convey hope. However, it is also important to be accurate. In the case of diseases, learn as much as you can about prognosis prior to the discussion and offer as much hope as possible. If there is any degree of uncertainty about the prognosis, don't make promises or offer unrealistic expectations. Even when delivering news about potentially life-ending illnesses, a caring statement such as, *"No matter what happens, we'll do everything we can to keep you comfortable"* is more authentic than promising false hope. In the case of HIV, it is critical to address prevailing myths about the virus. HIV is not a death sentence and can be well managed. Whenever possible, offer a reassuring statement that suggests that the teen is not alone and that you believe he will get through this: *"I have cared for [many/several] other youth with X and I have seen them get through this. I believe that you will also."*

12. *Continue to listen.* As the moments proceed, the youth will often reveal what he needs through his words or actions. Listening may be more important than anything you say. Listening reinforces that you are present. Listening conveys that you respect the youth as the expert on his own life. Listening allows you to serve as a sounding board as the adolescent facilitates his own progress.

13. *Explore how best to get ongoing support.* It is important before the youth leaves your presence that he has thought through who else can offer ongoing support. Ask directly, *"Who in your life can be most helpful now?"* That person does not have to be a parent, but ideally will be a supportive adult. If there is no accessible or responsible adult, then your continued presence becomes particularly important. In the case of bad news, particularly the kind that may (sadly) have stigma attached (eg, HIV), you should not push toward disclosure before the young person is ready.

14. *Assess for safety.* It is imperative that you ask directly if the young person feels safe. In the case of bad personal news, he may be considering self-harm. In the case of bad news about a friend or family members, particularly if it involved violence, the teen may be considering retaliation. In either case, safety becomes the top priority and, after a more thorough assessment, you might need to heighten the level of protection for the young person or report a threat to authorities. Privacy is no longer protected when a life is threatened.

15. *Create a follow-up plan.* In some case*s, you might refer* to a person more adept at the level of care the youth needs. Even in these cases, the adolescent should still have a follow-up plan to see you in a few days. This will reinforce that you are committed to the teen getting through this and not feeling alone. In a crisis situation, let the adolescent know that someone in your practice or agency is available at all times if the youth needs added support. If this is not the case, then make sure the young person has a hotline number to call if for some reason he cannot wait until morning. As important as it is to make yourself available for follow-up, it is even more vital not to overpromise. Many youth have experience with adults who have been inconsistent and unavailable; you do not want to be added to that list. Be clear and honest about your service and limitations. When you will try to make something happen but cannot guarantee the result, say just that.

14.1

■ The Debrief as a Standard Part of the Process

Witnessing pain takes a toll on us. No matter how many times you will shepherd young people through difficult times, it will continue to affect you. Debrief with colleagues both to process your own emotions and to incorporate "lessons learned" to be able to handle similar situations in the future.

■ Parents as Critical Allies

Ideally, parents will be the most supportive figures in their children's lives. However, they also experience grief, shock, and stigma. Those emotions may prevent them from giving their best performance. In addition, they may experience anger and guilt. The combination of anger and guilt are a toxic mixture, because, to alleviate their own sense of guilt, they may intensify their anger toward their teen. This may be particularly true in your presence because they are trying to communicate to you, the authority figure, *"This is not my fault."*

It is important, therefore, to break bad news to parents in a way that diminishes their guilt. Their presence alone enables you to do this.

■ Contributing to the World as a Healing Exercise

The following strategies are not recommended on the first day that bad news is delivered. Then, your goals are conveying accurate information, providing emotional support, and crisis management, if necessary. However, the follow-up visit may be the time to help the youth think about how to move forward in a way that allows them to improve the situation for someone else. In some cases, it may be something you suggest long after a teen has progressed on their own healing journey.

The technique may be helpful when the bad news involved loss of someone who the youth cared deeply about. People who experience grief often have no place to channel it, and can sometimes come up with very negative responses such as, *"I'll kill myself to be closer with my grandma,"* or *"They killed my brother; he's not around to get even, I will."* Instead, help the youth to take on a good deed or activity to honor the life of the loved one. *"Tell me about your grandma." "What were her dreams for you?" "Could you imagine making them come true to honor her life?"* or *"Tell me about your brother." What are the good things he brought to the world?" "How can you make his memory live on in a positive way?"* This technique is particularly useful when someone leaves behind a child or elderly relative to be cared for. *"Let's make sure your niece knows about your brother's sense of humor and how much he loved her. Could you imagine making her a storybook about him? Do you think you can watch out for her?"*

In the cases of teens whose bad news is about themselves, they may eventually benefit from sharing lessons learned with peers. It may help them to make more sense of why something happened to them. *"I guess it is my job to make sure this doesn't happen to other kids."* This strategy is not something to be pushed; it needs to follow disclosure. Rather, it remains an option that some youth may find healing. A sense of contribution is a core element of resilience. ▶ **5.1, 8.5**

●● Group Learning and Discussion ●●

Break into pairs and choose scenarios that match your professional settings from among the following and practice breaking the news to the young person. Alternatively, pick an actual situation and share it with your partner. Before you role-play, discuss how you might feel as the professional in each situation. That process will parallel the recommendation that in an actual situation you first consider your own reaction.

1. You are in a group home. Tyler is a 14-year-old boy who was removed from his home for parental neglect and school truancy. You just received a call that his 18-year-old brother was shot and killed.

2. You are a nurse practitioner who just received biopsy results on Lisa, a 16-year-old patient who reminds you of your niece. She had a long-standing enlarged lymph node, and, although you were very reassuring, you sent her to have it biopsied. She has cancer. After a preliminary discussion with an oncologist, you are reassured that her prognosis is good.

3. You work in a testing center, and Felipe, a 15-year-old boy, has tested positive for HIV.

4. You work in a residential setting that serves youth. You receive a call that 13-year-old Marita's mother was in a car crash and died. There is not a family member available nearby.

■ Suggested Reading

Leventown M; American Academy of Pediatrics Committee on Bioethics. Communicating with children and families: from everyday interactions to skill in conveying distressing information. *Pediatrics.* 2008;121(5):e1441–e1460. http://pediatrics.aappublications.org/content/121/5/e1441.full.html. Accessed June 25, 2013

■ Related Video Content

14.0 Among the Hardest Things We Do—Delivering Bad News. Ginsburg, Reirden, Arrington-Sanders, Garofalo, Hawkins, Pletcher.

14.1 Never Make Promises to Homeless and Marginalized Youth That You Cannot Keep. Hill.

5.1 Dealing With Grief by Living Life More Purposefully. Ginsburg.

8.5 Stress Management and Coping/Section 4/Making the World Better/Point 10: Contribute. Ginsburg.

9.3 Mindful Walking. Vo.

De-escalation and Crisis Management Strategies

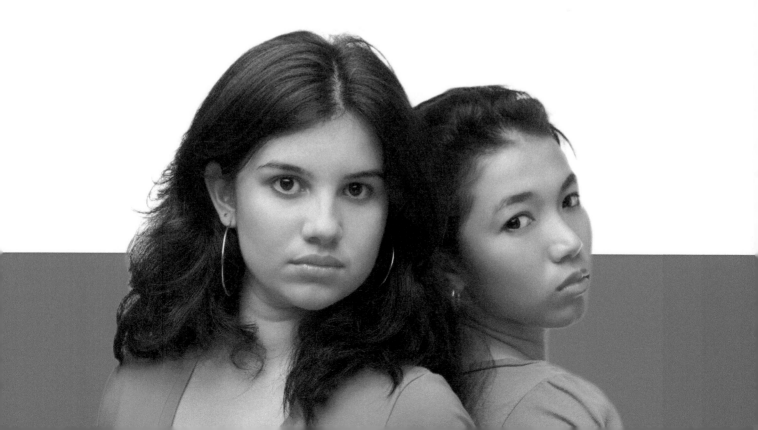

CHAPTER 15

De-escalation and Crisis Management When a Youth Is "Acting Out"

Cordella Hill, MSW
Hugh Organ, MS
Kenneth R. Ginsburg, MD, MS Ed, FAAP, FSAHM

 Related Video Content

15.0 De-escalation and Crisis Management: Wisdom and Strategies From Professionals Who Serve Youth Who Often Act Out Their Frustrations

■ Why This Matters

This text focuses on connecting with youth and reasoning with them in a shared decision-making process while engaging them to consider positive behavioral changes. In sharp contrast, during an acute crisis that may involve acting out, the only goals are safety and de-escalation. In fact, attempts at reasoning may be counter-productive because expecting an irrational youth to consider long-range outcomes or abstract concepts may enhance his feelings of incompetence and frustration, inadvertently magnifying the crisis.

> The actions necessary to de-escalate a rising crisis run counter to the fight or flight instincts we have to respond to stressful or threatening situations. Therefore, it is especially important to draw from a well thought out, practiced skill set.

The actions necessary to de-escalate a rising crisis run counter to the fight or flight instincts we have to respond to stressful or threatening situations. Therefore, it is especially important to draw from a well thought out, practiced skill set.

The overall goals of acute crisis management are to

1. Ensure immediate safety for the teen and others in the setting, including yourself.
2. Deescalate the situation.
3. Assess for the potential of ongoing harm to self or others.
4. Refer to appropriate resources.
5. Debrief with your colleagues to process emotions and learn from the episode.

■ Limitations of This Chapter

If you work in a youth crisis center or facility that serves youth with mental health challenges, you deserve an intensive training in crisis management. This chapter is designed to introduce concepts and broaden your repertoire; it does not substitute for formal professional development.

■ Safety First

Safety always comes first. It is optimal to be able to communicate with a person in acute crisis and resolve any outstanding issues. However, if there is any potential for physical harm, security or the police need to be involved, and you might have to consider physical and/or medical restraints. Appropriate use of restraints is beyond the scope of this chapter.

When considering safety, the following points may be helpful:

- Inform colleagues that you are entering a difficult situation before you enter the room, and have someone monitor the evolving scenario.
- Prior to entering the room, remove any necklaces, ties, or other objects from around your neck. (If someone cuts off your air supply, you cannot summon help.)
- Remove any religious or political symbols, as it is difficult to predict a reaction they might trigger.
- Keep the door open.
- Do not allow anything to be between you and the door.
- Do not stand between the youth and the door so that he does not feel trapped.
- Consider going in with another person. Depending on the situation, this may interfere with or enhance optimal communication, but it can be critical if there is a serious concern about safety.
- Never turn your back for any reason.

Quickly Assessing for Drug Use or Psychosis

It is important to quickly assess whether verbal de-escalation may help you address a crisis.

- If a person is psychotic, as indicated by his behavior being disconnected to reality, it is especially important to be calming and to use nonconfrontational body language. It is also especially important to remain nonjudgmental, but it may not be helpful to enter a verbal discussion.
- Similarly, if a person appears to be hallucinating, it may be dangerous to attempt to reach him, as his distorted sense of reality may paint you as antagonistic. Although youth under the influence of most drugs can be calmed, youth on PCP as well as some other hallucinogens, such as bath salts, may become more agitated with any attempts at communication. One telltale sign of PCP is horizontal, vertical, and rotatory nystagmus, as indicated by eyes making quick involuntary movements in all directions as they attempt to track an object.

Getting Rid of the Audience

A critical first step to de-escalation is to clear the area of any audience. Especially in the case of a conflict or a fight, a young person's need to perform for onlookers will make it much harder for her to back down or return to calm. Further, youth in crowds can intentionally inflame a situation.

Breaking Up a Fight

It is beyond the scope of this chapter to offer physical maneuvers that may help you to safely separate 2 aggressive parties. The wisest strategy is to remember that safety comes first and to involve police or security right away.

Below are some general rules.

1. First, attempt to stop the fight using a clear, stern, loud voice to demand the fight stop immediately.
2. Remove the crowd immediately.
3. Do not step into the middle of the fight.
4. If you have a prior relationship with either combatant, verbally redirect that combatant to leave the situation. If no prior relationship exists, then identify the least aggressive combatant and verbally redirect that person away from the situation.
5. If the combatants are not separating, create a loud distraction. When you gain their eye contact, demand that they separate.
6. Move combatants into 2 separate areas.
7. Do not ask, "Who started this?"
8. Do very little talking until the adrenalin surge appears to be subsiding, as judged by breathing returning to normal and the youth seeming less physically agitated.
9. Follow de-escalation strategies discussed elsewhere.

■ De-escalation

Absolute Respect

An irritable or agitated teen is acutely sensitive to being disrespected or feeling shamed. He needs to know that, even as we set limits, it comes from our caring and desire to protect him. Our challenge is to remain deeply respectful throughout our intervention and to treat him with full dignity, even in the extreme case where physical restraints are needed.

Anticipating a Problem

Your practice group should devise a plan to deal with adolescent crises before one is needed. Your decisions are more likely to be thoughtful than those made when on the receiving end of anger or emotional outbursts. Think about those issues likely to arise in your setting and develop strategies as a group ahead of time.

On any given day, the best de-escalation plans occur before a crisis strikes. If a youth seems angry at something that you did, apologize. If a youth feels frustrated and powerless, give a choice that allows her to regain a sense of power. If a teen feels frightened, reassure her that you will keep her safe. Notice signs of increasing anxiety, such as pacing, fidgeting, hand wringing, or withdrawal, and share that the young person seems upset or worried. Ask if there is anything you can do to be supportive. If stress is building, listen to the teen's concerns until she feels as if she has been fully heard. If it is clear that a crisis is at hand, consider referral to a crisis center or psychiatric emergency department in advance of escalation.

The Body Language of De-escalation

The young person in acute crisis is likely to be experiencing anxiety or anger, and may feel vulnerable to attack. Therefore, she is likely to be hypervigilant of any movement perceived to be potentially hostile. The first step of de-escalation is to reassure the youth that there is no imminent threat and, indeed, that your presence supports, rather than challenges, safety. Calming body language is critical in combination with verbal reassurance.

Your natural reaction to an impending challenge or threat is to have anxiety or to feel personally endangered. Therefore, your instincts will be telling you to either flee or take an offensive position yourself. First, control your breathing with deep slow breaths so that you will reverse the "fight or flight" response (see Chapter 8). Then, use reassuring "self-talk" to gain confidence that you are well prepared and are best able to handle the situation with your skill, rather than your physical power. Remind yourself that the hostility or fear is likely not directed at you. Even if it is directed toward you, then you are especially well positioned to de-escalate the situation with an apology for anything you might have done to cause offense. These thoughts and actions will control your instinctual biological reactions and may better allow your body to display the calm, yet controlled, demeanor needed to reassure the young person of safety.

It is important to give the agitated young person plenty of physical space. His or her "personal space" will be greater than normal. A hostile or frightened youth will be sensitive to any threat; therefore, movement into personal space can trigger alarm. This is particularly true if the youth has a history of trauma. It is best not to have any physical contact while the youth is agitated. If you extend a hand, make sure that your hands are clearly open. That will help the teen see that there is no weapon present and prevent your movement from being interpreted as if you are planning to grasp and control the arm. Similarly, keep your hands out of your pockets both to signal that you have no weapon and so that they are available for self-protection. A palms-up position illustrates that your desire is to serve rather than dominate.

Try to communicate reassurance and concern with your facial expression. Hopefully, your reassuring self-talk will allow you to avoid a countenance of fear. A smile may be viewed as insincere or can be misinterpreted as nervousness, a grimace, or as if you are minimizing the irritable youth's concerns. Eye contact is a sign of respect in most cultures. Remain at the same eye level as the youth. Try to stay seated, but if he needs to stand, rise to meet his eyes. Although eye contact is respectful, allow him to break his gaze and look away.

Next, position your body at an angle to the youth. A chest-to-chest position can send subconscious hostile messages and trigger instinctual expectations of an imminent attack. An angled position diminishes this sense while actually better positioning you to escape if necessary.

It is important to also watch the pace of your movements. Slow, methodical movements reinforce calm. Quick movements may give away your own anxiety. Further, any rapid movements can trigger anxiety or a defensive hostile reaction in a young person acutely sensitive to danger.

Listening

It is hard to find the perfect words to say when a person is frantic or acting out. The good news is that listening—the relative absence of words—is the key to de-escalation. Start by telling the young person that your goal is to listen to their feelings and concerns. Sit down or use other body language cues to demonstrate that you are not in a hurry. Silence can be an effective tool because it reinforces your intention to listen. If the young person continues to yell, you might consider saying in a calm even tone, *"I really want to hear you, and I'm having trouble hearing what you're telling me when you are talking this way. I am really here to listen, and I'm going to listen until you're done talking."*

A Few Words to Say…and What Not to Say

An acute crisis is not the time to help someone resolve multiple issues. It is not a time to argue or try to convince a teen of your viewpoint. Therefore, keep conversations simple and concrete, while avoiding any abstract complexity or lectures. A person in crisis cannot think abstractly. When your discussion is complex, you can inadvertently reinforce a sense of shame because of the teen's inability to grasp your points while she is in crisis mode. Once she has been calmed, you can consider facilitating her to develop and own her own solutions (see Chapter 12). Until she has reached that state of calm, which you can sense by the rate of her breathing, the cadence of her speech, and her posture, your words should be few, simple, reassuring, and calming. Avoid language that implies you understand what she is feeling or that belittles or negates her emotions. Don't say too much; instead focus on listening and use silence judiciously. Silence can trigger discussion as people tend to fill the void. Never interrupt while the youth is talking. When the teen is done talking, ask *"Is there anything else you'd like to tell me?"*

DON'T SAY	SAY INSTEAD
I understand.	Help me to understand.
I know how you feel.	I can't imagine how you feel.
Just calm down.	You seem angry. I'm here to listen so you can get your feelings out.
Just get over it.	After you work out your feelings, you're going to get through this.
You're making a big deal out of nothing.	This seems so important to you.
You're always causing trouble here and that's not acceptable.	This place has to feel safe for everyone, including you.
I agree.	I hear you.
It sounds like he was totally wrong.	I hear what you are saying. I'll get to the bottom of this.
Don't have an attitude with me, I'm here to help you.	You really seem frustrated. I definitely want to hear everything you have to say, and we're going to figure this out together.
You're always causing trouble.	You've come so far. I've been so proud of you because _____. You're having a tough day. I have confidence you'll get through this.

Tone of Voice

Verbal communication is more than about what you say; it is also about how you say it. Your tone and cadence easily give away your anxiety or anger. Your volume suggests whether you wish to dominate or control. A loud volume can be interpreted as an attempt to dampen another's voice. Softer speech suggests you are listening with no intent of diminishing the other's ability to express their thoughts and feelings. In fact, as a person raises their voice, lower yours. As their cadence increases, slow yours. This way you can show with your body language, your words, and how those words are expressed that your goal is to listen. A young person who feels heard will often be able to return to a state of calm.

Offering an Apology

If a young person is angry with you, an apology can go a long way. If you may have done something wrong, a heartfelt apology is warranted. Ideally, an apology should be spontaneously given prior to escalation, because it can prevent the cycle of anger from the beginning. An apologetic statement does not have to be an admission of guilt, rather it is used to acknowledge someone's feelings and begin to redress a perceived wrong. You can always choose to apologize for someone's experience: *"I am sorry for how that felt to you"* or *"I am sorry for how my words made you angry."*

Avoid Defensiveness and Answer All Questions Respectfully

Even if the anger or insults are directed at you, it is critical to remember they are rarely really about you. Do not feel the need to defend yourself or any of your colleagues from insults, curses, or denigration about their roles. Answer all questions that are genuinely seeking information no matter the tone in which they are asked, because the information may defuse the crisis. Do not feel the need to respond to questions that feel abusive, and that are not really calling for information (eg, *"Why does everyone here suck?"*). Such a question needs neither a response nor defensiveness.

Giving Something

A person in crisis may make unreasonable or irrational demands. Even if their request is appropriate, you still may not be able to fulfill it. In order to avoid escalation, it can be strategic to offer something else. You might say, *"I'm sorry but I don't think I'll be able to _____, but I think I will be able to _____."* Even if the young person does not make a request, it is still nice to offer something because it places you in the role of caregiver. Consider saying, *"Do you want me to get you some water/juice/a snack while we talk?"* (Only offer a physical object, even a snack, as the situation is calming. Otherwise, it can be thrown at you.) Depending on the circumstance, you might consider stating, *"I'm wondering if I was able to _____, whether that would help. What do you think?"* It can also be effective to offer the youth the opportunity to choose between different appropriate choices because choices give teens a sense of control, and few things can restore calm like a sense of control.

Offering Clear Boundaries

Even amidst a crisis, do not be afraid to explain limits and rules in an authoritative, firm tone. It actually may make the teen feel safer to know that you need to maintain safety for everyone and that he will be contained. It also offers him a face-saving way to de-escalate when you respectfully, but clearly, demand appropriate behavior. Offer choices in which both alternatives are reasonable (eg, *"Would you like to continue our discussion now or would you prefer to come back later when you have had a chance to think things through?"*). It is possible to empathize fully with a feeling without validating a behavior (eg, *"I understand that you have a really good reason to feel frustrated, even angry, but it is not okay for you to threaten me or any of the other youth."*).

■ Assessing Ongoing Risk

After de-escalating the acute crisis, you need to determine the young person's risk for harm to self or others. If the youth does express suicidal or homicidal intent, it becomes both your ethical and legal obligation to protect the teen, and you may not keep the information confidential.

Tell the young person that you are glad that she was able to express herself and that although she seems to feel better, you want to make sure she remains safe. Then ask directly whether you have to worry about the possibility of her hurting herself or someone else. Explore the degree of likelihood of a further incident by asking whether a plan exists and ascertaining the details of that plan. Always err toward caution, and do not assume the teen is just blowing off steam.

■ Referral

The immediacy and type of referral depends on whether the situation was able to be calmed and whether your assessment revealed an imminent risk. If you were not able to de-escalate the episode, you may need to involve the police or a mobile crisis team. If the crisis is de-escalated, but the teen remains at imminent risk, then he or she requires immediate psychiatric evaluation. If there is no imminent risk, then your challenge is to persuade the young person that he is deserving of further ongoing support. It may be that the youth will not be prepared to transition to mental health care, in which case your goal should be to maintain a relationship so you can continue to guide him, reassess his need in the future, and continue to build trust so that you can readdress the need for mental health care later.

■ Debrief

It is important to debrief with colleagues or a supervisor after a major episode. First, it is important to process your own emotions to relieve some of your stress. Don't be surprised, even if you were the model of collection in the midst of a crisis, if your fears come out after calm is restored. A debrief is also a good time to consider quality improvement: What was done well? What could have been handled better? How could the response be improved the next time a crisis presents? Perhaps most importantly, when we debrief as a group, it allows the entire team to learn from a situation that may only have involved 1 or 2 people.

●● Group Learning and Discussion ●●

Preparing a Practice for a Potential Episode
- What are the kinds of crises likely to present in our setting?
- What plans do we have in place to ensure the safety of our staff and teens in crisis, as well as other teens and families?
- Is security easily accessible? Could we easily signal distress to our colleagues such that a staff member not directly involved would know when and how to summon security?
- Does everyone know to eliminate the audience first, to ensure their safety and decrease the likelihood they will inflame the situation?
- What steps does a staff member need to take before entering a room to ensure his or her own safety?
- Review key elements of a nonconfrontational body language.
- Review key points about what to say and what not to say in a potentially explosive situation.
- Discuss the strategic reasons to apologize to an angry youth.

The Debrief: Discussion Questions for After an Episode
- Were there any indications that the teen was moving toward a crisis?
- Is there anything that we could have done to have prevented the escalation?
- Is there anything we did that upset the teen? Was it avoidable?
- Assuming that we were verbally attacked or insulted, or one of our colleagues was defamed, how did that affect us emotionally?
- How did it feel to see a youth in that much pain?
- Did we do everything we could to ensure safety first? Let's review those steps.
- Did the issue get resolved adequately? If not, where do we stand now? If yes, what seemed to have made the difference? What allowed the young person to calm down?
- Are there any lessons learned that we have to put into place to make us better prepared for the next incident?

■ Suggested Reading

Couvillon M, Peterson RL, Ryan JB, Scheuermann B, Stegall J. A review of crisis intervention training programs for schools. TEACHING Except Child. 2010;42(5):6–17

Crisis Prevention Institute. CPI Nonviolent Crisis Intervention Training Program. De-escalation Techniques. http://www.crisisprevention.com/Resources/Knowledge-Base/De-escalation-Tips/De-escalation-Techniques. Accessed September 4, 2013

Skolnik-Acker E, Committee for the Study and Prevention of Violence Against Social Workers, National Association of Social Workers, Massachusetts Chapter. Verbal De-escalation Techniques for Defusing or Talking Down an Explosive Situation. http://www.naswma.org/displaycommon. cfm?an=1&subarticlenbr=520. Accessed September 4, 2013

■ Related Video Content

15.0 De-escalation and Crisis Management: Wisdom and Strategies From Professionals Who Serve Youth Who Often Act Out Their Frustrations. Youth-serving agencies.

15.1 De-escalation if Someone Wants to Leave to "Get Even." Covenant House.

15.2 Why Youth Act Out…and What They Really Need. YouthBuild youth.

15.3 Trauma-Informed Practice: Working With Youth Who Have Suffered Adverse Experiences. El Centro staff, Covenant House staff.

■ Related Web Sites

If your group is interested in formal training in nonviolent de-escalation, below are reputable programs that offer staff professional development sessions.

CPI Nonviolent Crisis Intervention Training
www.crisisprevention.com

Handle With Care Behavior Management System
http://handlewithcare.com

Index

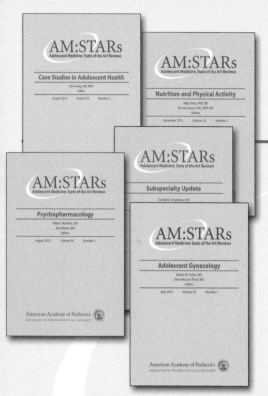

AM:STARs

Adolescent Medicine: State of the Art Reviews

Adolescent Medicine: State of the Art Reviews is the official publication of the AAP Section on Adolescent Health. Published 3 times per year, it offers adolescent medicine specialists and other primary care physicians who treat adolescents timely information on all matters relating to adolescent health and wellness. Each issue centers on a specific topic area with expert advice.

Adolescent Medicine: State of the Art Reviews is a rolling subscription. Annual 3-edition subscription begins with the next available issue.

SUB1006
Price: $124.95   Member Price: $114.95   Student Price: $63   Institutions: $174.95

Upcoming Publication Schedule

Young Adult Health
December 2013
Volume 24, Issue 3
Editors: David Rosen, MD, MPH
Alain Joffe, MD, MPH

Substance Use and Abuse by Adolescents
April 2014
Volume 25, Issue 1
Editors: Robert Brown, MD
Sheryl Ryan, MD

Hot Topics in Adolescent Medicine
August 2014
Volume 25, Issue 2
Editors: Cynthia Holland-Hall, MD
Paula Braverman, MD

AM:STARs back issues
Price: $59.95 Member Price: $54.95

Nutrition and Physical Activity
Editors: Mary Story, PhD, RD
Nicole Larson, PhD, MPH, RD
MA0595   ISBN: 978-1-58110-603-9
eISBN: 978-1-58110-783-8

Subspecialty Update
Editor: Donald E. Greydanus, MD
MA0648   ISBN: 978-1-58110-749-4
eISBN: 978-1-58110-807-1

Current Psychopharmacology for Psychiatric Disorders in Adolescents
Editors: Robert L. Hendren, DO
Alya Reeve, MD, MPH
MA0649   ISBN: 978-1-58110-750-0

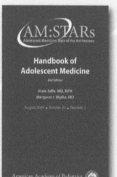

Handbook of Adolescent Medicine, 2nd Edition

Editors: Alain Joffe, MD, MPH
Margaret J. Blythe, MD

Devoted to issues that adolescent medicine specialists are likely to encounter on any given day, it includes material gathered from a variety of sources, including textbooks, classic review articles, insights of colleagues, and more. Find answers fast with this valuable quick reference guide.

Softcover, 2009
MA0479
ISBN: 978-1-58110-334-2
eISBN: 978-1-58110-405-9
Price: $59.95   Member Price: $54.95

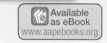
Available as eBook
www.aapebooks.org

For a complete list of **AM:STARs** back issues in print and eBook, visit **www.aap.org/bookstore.**

Key AAP resources for adolescent health professionals

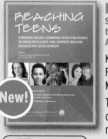

New!

Reaching Teens
Strength-Based Communication Strategies to Build Resilience and Support Healthy Adolescent Development

Kenneth R. Ginsburg, MD, MS Ed, FAAP, FSAHM, and Sara B. Kinsman, MD, PhD

This all-new multimedia resource combines text and video to show how recognizing, reinforcing, and building on inherent strengths can engage today's teens.

Available as eBook
www.aapebooks.org

MA0647
ISBN: 978-1-58110-748-7
eISBN: 978-1-58110-834-7
Price: $149.95   Member Price: $139.95

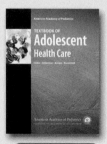

AAP Textbook of Adolescent Health Care

Editor in Chief:
Martin M. Fisher, MD, FAAP
Coeditors:
Elizabeth M. Alderman, MD, FAAP
Richard E. Kreipe, MD, FAAP
Walter D. Rosenfeld, MD, FAAP

Trustworthy guidance spanning every aspect of adolescent health care.

Available as eBook
www.aapebooks.org

MA0403
ISBN: 978-1-58110-269-7
eISBN: 978-1-58110-565-0
Price: $169.95   Member Price: $154.95

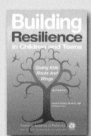

Building Resilience in Children and Teens: Giving Kids Roots and Wings

Kenneth R. Ginsburg, MD, MS Ed, FAAP, FSAHM, With Martha M. Jablow

CB0065
ISBN: 978-1-58110-551-3
eISBN: 978-1-58110-619-0
Price: $15.95
Member Price: $15.95

Available as eBook
www.aapebooks.org

To order these adolescent resources, visit the AAP Bookstore at **www.aap.org/bookstore.**

American Academy of Pediatrics
DEDICATED TO THE HEALTH OF ALL CHILDREN™